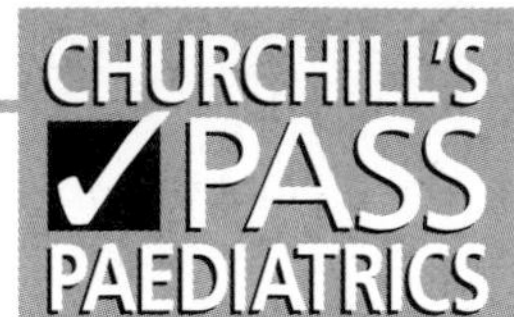

Paediatric Grey Cases for the MRCPCH

Commissioning Editor: Ellen Green
Project Development Manager: Janice Urquhart
Project Manager: Nancy Arnott
Design direction: Judith Wright

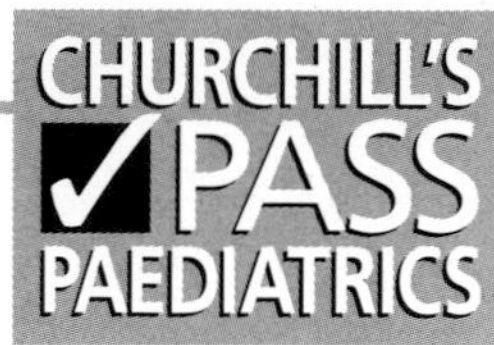

Paediatric Grey Cases for the MRCPCH

Alan C. Fenton
MD FRCPCH MRCP(UK)
Consultant Paediatrician,
Royal Victoria Infirmary,
Newcastle upon Tyne, UK

Sean B. Ainsworth
MB ChB MRCP(UK) MRCPCH DCH
Specialist Registrar in Paediatrics,
Royal Victoria Infirmary,
Newcastle upon Tyne, UK

Nicholas D. Plant
MB BCh FRCP FRCPCH
Consultant Paediatric Nephrologist,
Royal Victoria Infirmary,
Newcastle upon Tyne, UK

Paraic J. McGrogan
MB ChB MRCP MRCPCH
Clinical Research Fellow,
Sir James Spence Institute of Child Health, Royal Victoria Infirmary,
Newcastle upon Tyne, UK

David W. A. Milligan
MB BS DCH FRCP FRCPCH BA
Consultant Paediatrician,
Royal Victoria Infirmary,
Newcastle upon Tyne, UK

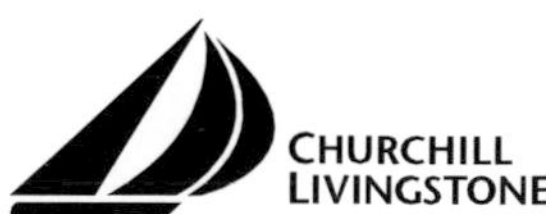

EDINBURGH LONDON NEW YORK OXFORD PHILADELPHIA ST LOUIS SYDNEY TORONTO 2002

CHURCHILL LIVINGSTONE
An imprint of Elsevier Limited

First published 2002
Reprinted 2003, 2004, 2005

ISBN 0 443 06444 X

British Library Cataloguing in Publication Data
A catalogue record for this book is available from the British Library

Library of Congress Cataloguing in Publication Data
A catalogue record for this book is available from the Library of Congress

Note
Medical knowledge is constantly changing. As new information becomes available, changes in treatment, procedures, equipment and the use of drugs become necessary. The editors, contributor and the publishers have taken care to ensure that the information given in this text is accurate and up to date. However, readers are strongly advised to confirm that the information, especially with regard to drug usage, complies with the latest legislation and standards of practice.

The Publisher

The publisher's policy is to use **paper manufactured from sustainable forests**

Printed in China
C/04

Contents

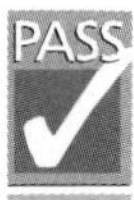

Preface

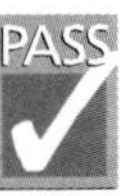

The MRCPCH Part II examination consists of written and clinical sections. This book is intended to help candidates prepare for the 'grey case' section of the written examination and contains 100 'grey cases' divided into 20 papers. Many of the cases are composites of history, examination and clinical material such as X-rays, photographs and ECGs. One or two of the 'diagnoses' occur in several of the papers so that you will be unable to discount them as an answer simply because they have already appeared.

It is planned to increase the number of questions in this section of the examination by using shorter questions and asking candidates to select 'best fit' answers. We would encourage you to approach these questions as you would in 'real life' and we have included an extended list of potential investigations in some of the answers.

We suggest that each paper be completed in its entirety before the answers are checked. The time allowed for this section in the examination is 55 minutes. In keeping with the real examination, normal ranges are not given for results of standard investigations but are included for more unusual tests.

A. C. F. 2001
S. B. A.
N. D. P.
P. J. McG.
D. W. A. M

Acknowledgements

We would like to acknowledge our many colleagues who have contributed to this project, in particular Andrew Crisp, Tim Cheetham, Nick Embleton, Sue Glass, Neil Hopper, Andrew Morris, Nadeem Moghal, Chris O'Brien, Martin Smith and John O'Sullivan.

Paper 1 *Questions*

QUESTION 1.1

A 12-year-old girl is referred with worsening control of her asthma. This had been diagnosed at the age of 6 years and had initially responded to appropriate doses of inhaled steroids and bronchodilators. Over the preceding 12 months she had experienced severe exertional dyspnoea with wheeze following minimal exercise and this had not responded to increases in her inhaled steroids or the introduction of long-acting bronchodilators. Her GP had also tried a course of oral steroids with minimal improvement. There was no apparent allergic component to her symptoms. She was troubled a great deal by a non-productive cough, although her mother felt it was much less of a problem at night. She was missing a great deal of school on account of the cough. On examination she looks well but has a dry-sounding intermittent cough. Her height is on the 75th centile and her weight on the 99th. Chest examination is entirely unremarkable. Her inhaler technique is good and her peak flow on the 25th centile for her height. A chest radiograph is normal.

1. Suggest the most likely diagnosis.
2. Give two tests you would use to investigate this girl further.

QUESTION 1.2

A 6-week-old male infant presents with a short history of irritability, fever, vomiting and loose stools. He was the first-born child to healthy unrelated parents. Pregnancy was normal and he had been well until the day of presentation. On examination the infant is clearly irritable, has a temperature of 39.8°C, is mottled and cold peripherally (capillary refill 6 seconds), has a pulse rate of 180/min but is normotensive. His anterior fontanelle is full. His umbilicus is not inflamed and the cord is dry and clean.

Haemoglobin	13.6 g/dl
White cell count	$32 \times 10^9/l$
Platelets	$98 \times 10^9/l$.

1. List four other investigations that are warranted.
2. What is your initial therapy?

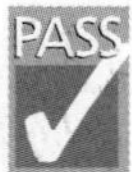

3. What is the immediate diagnosis?
4. What is the underlying disorder?

QUESTION 1.3

A 2-year-old boy attended with a relapse of steroid-sensitive nephrotic syndrome. He had been diagnosed at 10 months of age when he was noted to be oedematous with proteinuria on dipstick testing of an afternoon urine sample. Before his diagnosis he had failed to thrive and experienced intermittent vomiting and diarrhoea. At presentation he was commenced on high-dose oral prednisolone and his oedema settled within 3 weeks.

After his initial response to steroids he was well until prednisolone was discontinued after 2 months. He then became more irritable, experienced abdominal pain, diarrhoea and began to vomit again. His oedema returned and high-dose prednisolone was restarted. His symptoms resolved. He had three further episodes of oedema, preceded by diarrhoea, which all responded to steroids.

His growth chart showed episodes of poor weight gain when not taking prednisolone and consistently poor linear growth since before his diagnosis. He had an unremarkable past medical history but there was a family history of atopy and ischaemic heart disease.

Haemoglobin	9.2 g/dl
White cell count	$5.7 \times 10^9/l$
Platelets	$196 \times 10^9/l$
MCV	62 fl
Serum ferritin	6 ng/ml (normal 10–140 ng/ml)
Serum sodium	142 mmol/l
Serum potassium	4.4 mmol/l
Serum creatinine	33 μmol/l
Serum total calcium	2.35 mmol/l
Serum albumin	20 g/l

1. Give three further important investigations in this patient.
2. What is the appropriate next treatment?

QUESTION 1.4

A 14-year-old girl is admitted to the surgical ward with suspected appendicitis. She has had a 4-month history of intermittent lower abdominal pain. In the last 3 days she has had progressively more severe pain associated with difficulty in micturition and dribbling. As a 3-year-old she had a proven urinary tract infection. Investigations at that time included ultrasound of her renal tract and a DMSA scan, both of which were normal. She had been commenced on pizotifen for possible abdominal migraine two months previously. On systemic inquiry, she has regular bowel actions, no dysuria or loin pain and has not had her menarche.

On examination, she is afebrile. Her height and weight are both on the 75th centile. She has a soft non-tender goitre. Breast development is Tanner stage 5 and pubic hair stage 4.

Her BP is 100/65 mmHg. Abdominal examination reveals a suprapubic mass. Spinal examination is entirely normal.

Haemoglobin	10.9 g/dl
White cell count	9.3×10^9/l
Neutrophils	4.5×10^9/l
Lymphocytes	4.0×10^9/l
Platelets	356×10^9/l
Blood film	normal
Pregnancy test	negative
Urine microscopy	normal
Thyroid function tests	normal

1. List one immediate action.
2. What investigation would you carry out?
3. What is the diagnosis?
4. List three complications of this problem.

QUESTION 1.5

A female infant was born at term weighing 2890 g after a mid-cavity forceps delivery to a 34-year-old mother who had one previous healthy child. Apgar scores were 6 at 1 minute and 9 at 5 minutes. The infant was transferred to the postnatal ward with her mother and was discharged home breast feeding 12 hours later. At 5 days of age she was re-admitted because she was failing to feed and had started to vomit. Her mother said that, compared with her first child, this baby seemed difficult to satisfy. For the preceding 24 hours she had been more sleepy than usual and had been passing less urine.

On examination she was conscious but a little irritable and drowsy and weighed 2500 g. She was icteric. Her rectal temperature was 39°C. Her anterior fontanelle was slightly depressed and her heart rate was 150/min. Clinical examination was otherwise unremarkable. Following investigations she was started on antibiotics.

Haemoglobin	17.2 g/dl
Packed cell volume	55%
White cell count	19×10^9/l
Neutrophils	12×10^9/l
Platelets	180×10^9/l
Serum sodium	174 mmol/l
Serum potassium	5.2 mmol/l
Serum chloride	102 mmol/l
Serum urea	10 mmol/l
Serum creatinine	59 μmol/l
CSF	clear and colourless, no cells or organisms
CSF protein	0.6 g/l
CSF glucose	4.0 mmol/l

1. What is the most likely diagnosis?

Paper 1
Answers

1

ANSWER 1.1

1. Vocal cord dysfunction ('posterior chink' disorder)
2. Exercise stress test with pre- and post-exercise pulmonary function testing
   Upper airway endoscopy

This girl's symptoms are disproportionate to her signs and this, combined with school avoidance, suggests a 'somatiform' origin for the problem. Vocal cord dysfunction results in inappropriate approximation of the cords during inspiration, resulting in shortness of breath. Attacks may be precipitated by stress or exercise and be accompanied by wheeze; this particular patient had co-existent asthma. Stridor (inspiratory, expiratory and biphasic) occurs in up to 83% of cases. Spirometry may demonstrate flattening of the inspiratory portion of the flow volume curve, suggesting extrathoracic obstruction. Endoscopy may demonstrate adduction of the cords on inspiration leaving a diamond-shaped chink in the glottic aperture posteriorly. Treatment requires a multi-disciplinary approach including speech therapy for laryngeal relaxation techniques.

Other possible causes for this type of presentation include gastro-oesophageal reflux with aspiration, chronic sinusitis with post-nasal drip, vocal cord paralysis and laryngeal tumours.

ANSWER 1.2

1. Blood culture
   Urine culture
   Chest radiograph
   Lumbar puncture
2. Fluid resuscitation
   Broad-spectrum antibiotics (most commonly used are cefotaxime and ampicillin)
3. Late-onset neonatal sepsis ± meningitis
4. Adhesive glycoprotein molecule deficiency

Adhesive glycoprotein deficiency leads to a profound immunodeficiency affecting neutrophils, monocytes and some lymphocytes. There is markedly affected

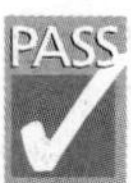

chemotaxis, adherence and phagocytosis. It is autosomal recessive. Affected infants present in the first few weeks with delayed cord separation and marked susceptibility to superficial and invasive pyogenic bacterial infection. Management consists of prophylactic antibiotics for moderate forms, progressing to bone marrow transplant for severe forms. Death is usual in the severe forms unless a bone marrow transplant can be performed.

ANSWER 1.3

1. Plasma anti-endomysial antibodies
   Jejunal biopsy
   Early morning urinary protein/creatinine ratio
2. Gluten-free diet
   Oral iron

This patient's coeliac disease was incorrectly diagnosed as steroid-sensitive nephrotic syndrome. During his first presentation a urine sample voided in the afternoon was assessed for protein using a dipstick. It revealed excess protein, consistent with the normal level of orthostatic proteinuria. His hypoalbuminaemia and oedema related to his underlying gluten enteropathy, which responded partially to treatment with oral steroids, a well-recognised phenomenon. Against a diagnosis of nephrosis is his age at presentation, a history of recurrent gastrointestinal symptoms (although abdominal pain may be a feature of hypovolaemia, peritonitis or pancreatitis during nephrotic relapses), poor height gain before presentation, and iron-deficiency anaemia.

ANSWER 1.4

1. Urinary catheterisation
2. Pelvic ultrasound
3. Haematocolpos
4. Urinary retention
   Endometriosis
   Pyohaematocolpos

This girl presents with primary amenorrhoea and secondary sex characteristics. A concealed pregnancy needs to be excluded, even before menarche. Imperforate hymen will present either at birth as a mucocolpos or at the time of menarche with the development of a haematocolpos. The symptoms will include cyclic pain, a pelvic mass, urinary retention and often a bulging hymen. Ultrasound will confirm the diagnosis. Treatment is incision of the membrane and drainage of the blood.

ANSWER 1.5

1. Dehydration and fever resulting from inadequate intake of concentrated breast milk

The cause of this baby's illness was dehydration resulting from a low water intake from his mother, whose breast milk was found to have a serum sodium concentration of 50 mmol/l, more than three times the normal value. As breast milk volume decreases it becomes more concentrated. The combination resulted in the hypernatraemic dehydration picture seen in this baby. Fever is a common accompanying feature. Non-accidental poisoning should always be considered in this situation, although this is unlikely when the chloride level is elevated less than the sodium (as in this baby) and when there is evidence of fluid loss rather than gain.

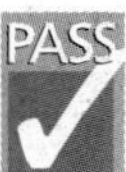

Paper 2 *Questions*

2

QUESTION 2.1

A 13-year-old boy is referred by his GP with obesity. He was born at term after an uneventful pregnancy and delivery and was well until the age of 3 years when he suffered a skull fracture as a result of a fall. He developed epilepsy (generalised tonic–clonic seizures) at 10 years of age, well controlled on sodium valproate. His school performance was said to be poor. On examination his weight is 58 kg (90th centile) and his height 146 cm (10th centile); both his father's and his brother's heights were around the 95th centile with appropriate weights, but his mother's height was < 3rd centile. She was said to have had difficulty in conceiving. In view of his obesity, thyroid function tests were performed with the following results:

TSH	11 mU/l (normal 0.3–4.5 mU/l)
T_4	9 pmol/l (normal 10–26 pmol/l)
Free T_3	2 nmol/l (normal 1–3 nmol/l)
Thyroid antibody screen	negative

1. What investigations would you perform next? List three.
2. Suggest a cause for his problems.

QUESTION 2.2

A 5-year-old boy was unwell with a viral illness 7 days ago. This morning he awoke complaining of seeing double and when he stood up he was unsteady on his feet. His GP referred him to hospital. On examination he is unable to gaze upwards, has a mild ptosis and left-sided facial weakness. He has mild weakness in both legs and lower limb reflexes are markedly diminished. When asked to walk he is unsteady and cannot stand straight. Fundoscopy is normal, and there is no sensory deficit.

1. What is the diagnosis?
2. How would you confirm this?
3. What is the treatment?
4. What is the eventual prognosis?

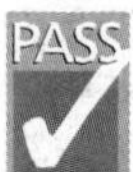

QUESTION 2.3

A 7-week-old male infant was referred for assessment of possible fits. He was delivered by elective lower segment Caesarean section at 39 weeks. He weighed 3450 g and needed resuscitation but was transferred to the postnatal ward. He was bottle-fed and took milk vigorously. At 5 days of age he was said to be 'difficult to settle' and 'colicky'. He posseted frequently and was in considerable discomfort after feeds. He cried excessively and exhibited abnormal head movements at these times. His health visitor felt that the movements might be neurological in origin. His parents described him as 'irritable'. He continued to feed voraciously throughout. His weight gain was poor. There was a strong family history of epilepsy.

At referral his weight was below the 3rd centile. No specific abnormalities were found on examination and his development appeared to be normal. Fundoscopy was normal. Following a feed he became distressed and upset. During this time he repetitively turned his neck to the right until his chin rested on his right clavicle. These dystonic movements continued for a few minutes. Neurological examination immediately following this episode was normal.

Serum sodium	136 mmol/l
Serum potassium	3.4 mmol/l
Serum urea	6.2 mmol/l
Serum creatinine	36 µmol/l
Serum bicarbonate	18 mmol/l
Blood glucose	4.7 mmol/l
Plasma ammonia	45 µmol/l (normal 21–50 µmol/l)
Prothrombin time	12 s (control 11–15 s)
Activated partial thromboplastin time	27 s (control 24–35 s)
Fibrinogen	2.1 g/l (normal 1.5–4.0 g/l)
Urinary amino-acid screen	normal
Urinary toxicology screen	normal

1. What is this condition known as?
2. What is the underlying problem?
3. How is this confirmed?

QUESTION 2.4

A 24-day-old male infant is referred with prolonged jaundice. He is breastfed. His birth weight was 3400 g and on admission he weighs 3800 g. He is the fourth child of non-consangineous parents. His two sisters (aged 8 years and 5 years) are both well. His brother, who is 2 years old, is under investigation for gross motor delay. On examination, he is non-dysmorphic and afebrile. Clinical examination is unremarkable. A soft liver edge 1 cm below the costal margin is noted. His stools are pigmented.

Haemoglobin	11.2 g/dl
White cell count	$5.7 \times 10^9/l$

Platelets	441×10^9/l
Total serum bilirubin	127 μmol/l
Conjugated bilirubin	13 μmol/l
Alanine transaminase	132 IU/l (normal 2–53 IU/l)
Gamma glutamyl transferase	30 IU/l (normal 5–55 IU/l)
Prothrombin time	15.1 s (control 11–15 s)
Activated partial thromboplastin time	32.0 s (control 24–35 s)
Thyroid function tests	normal
Alpha-1-antitryspin phenotype	MM
Sweat chloride	29 mmol/100 g

No action is taken at the time. He failed to reattend until 1 year of age when his health visitor reorganised the appointment. At 1 year his weight is 12.3 kg. Abdominal examination is unremarkable.

Total serum bilirubin	23 μmol/l
Conjugated bilirubin	3 μmol/l
Alanine transaminase	344 IU/l
Gamma glutamyl transferase	27 IU/l
Prothrombin time	12.0 s
Activated partial thromboplastin time	29.2 s
Serum albumin	41 g/l

1. What two investigations would you carry out?
2. What is the diagnosis?
3. What is the genetic inheritance of this disease?

QUESTION 2.5

An 11-month-old boy was brought to clinic by his parents with a story of intermittent cough and wheeze. He had been well in the past apart from recurrent vomiting, which had improved on Gaviscon. About 4 months previously he had a paroxysm of coughing whilst he was playing on the floor in the sitting room. Since then the coughing had persisted intermittently and he had been wheezing. He was otherwise well and was growing and developing normally. There was a history of asthma and hay fever on the father's side of the family and his mother's sister had diabetes. The remainder of the family (two older sisters) and his mother were well.

On examination he was cheerful and well but intermittently had a brief spasm of coughing. There was some subcostal recession but breathing was not unduly laboured. There was a suggestion of a prolonged expiratory phase. Auscultation revealed diffuse low-pitched expiratory and some inspiratory rhonchi and air entry appeared reduced on the right. Clinical examination was otherwise unremarkable.

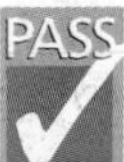

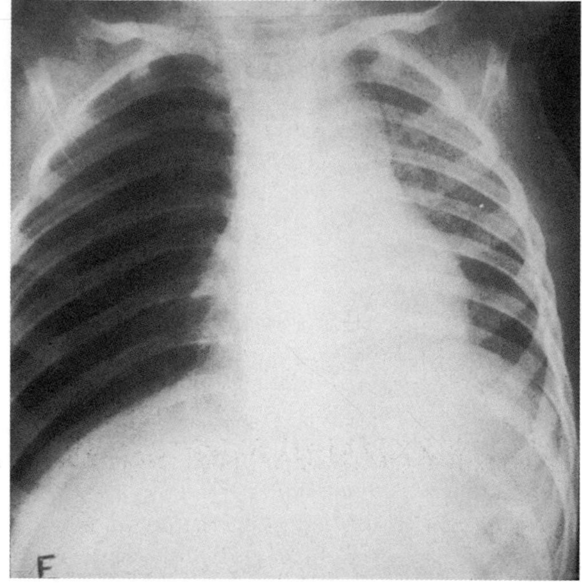

Fig. 2.1

A chest radiograph was performed (Fig. 2.1)

1. What does the radiograph show? List three features.
2. Give two clinical observations that might help elucidate the cause.

Paper 2
Answers

2

ANSWER 2.1

1. Serum calcium
   Serum phosphate
   Serum parathormone
2. Pseudohypoparathyroidism

This boy has a raised TSH in the presence of normal thyroid function. This may represent a 'compensated' hypothyroidism but the presence of short stature, obesity and poor school performance suggest pseudohypoparathyroidism. The diagnosis is supported by the maternal phenotype and difficulty in conceiving. The clinical features resemble those of hypoparathyroidism but the cause is renal resistance of target tissues to parathormone rather than simple lack of hormone.

Pseudohypoparathyroidism results from the loss of a trimeric guanine nucleotide-binding protein (G-protein) subunit that relays signals initiated by hormones. The G-protein subunit is common to many hormone receptors, hence the rise in TSH and the maternal history of difficulty in conceiving. It is likely that his mother has hypergonadotrophic hypogonadism as ovarian receptors are also affected. The range of clinical features seen in hypoparathyroidism can also be present in some (but not all) patients with pseudohypoparathyroidism; this clinical and biological heterogeneity is explained by the numerous molecular defects that can give rise to resistance to parathormone. Inheritance is mostly autosomal dominant (with phenotypic variability); maternal inheritance is associated with biochemical abnormalities in addition to the phenotypic features.

ANSWER 2.2

1. Miller Fisher syndrome (benign variant of Guillain–Barré syndrome)
2. Lumbar puncture and CSF examination for cells (pleocytosis) and protein estimation (elevated)
3. Supportive – physiotherapy to affected limbs
4. Good – the condition is self-resolving and recovery begins 2–4 weeks after onset of ataxia, with complete resolution by 6 months

Miller Fisher syndrome is a benign variant of Guillain–Barré syndrome. It affects young children (Guillain–Barré affects older children and adults) and, unlike Guillain–Barré syndrome, is thought to affect both central and peripheral nervous systems. A viral prodrome occurs 5–10 days before onset of acute ataxia in 50% of cases. Features of Miller Fisher syndrome include truncal ataxia (limbs may also be affected), areflexia, lower motor weakness of limbs and sometimes face. Ocular manifestations can occur and include ophthalmoplegia, paralysis of vertical gaze (upward gaze is affected more than downward), dissociated nystagmus, most marked in the abducting eye and ptosis. Guillain–Barré syndrome is the most common peripheral neuropathy of childhood. It presents mainly as a bilateral flaccid weakness with occasional paraesthesia and altered sensation. Reflexes are markedly reduced and plantars are flexor. Ocular involvement is rare in Guillain–Barré syndrome.

ANSWER 2.3

1. Sandifer's syndrome
2. Gastro-oesophageal reflux
3. Oesophageal pH study
   Contrast swallow

Sandifer's syndrome is the association between abnormal head posturing and gastro-oesophageal reflux. Such movements usually involve tilting and/or turning the head to one side and may also affect the upper body. They are postulated to reduce the pain associated with gastro-oesophageal reflux, protect the upper airway, improve oesophageal peristalsis and promote acid clearance from the distal oesophagus. The posturing can be mistaken for atypical seizures, dystonia or torticollis. The diagnosis of Sandifer's syndrome is made clinically in a child in whom gastro-oesophageal reflux has been confirmed on oesophageal pH monitoring. The movements resolve with treatment of the reflux.

ANSWER 2.4

1. Creatinine kinase levels
   Alanine transaminase isoenzymes
2. Duchenne muscular dystrophy
3. X-linked recessive

Alanine tramsaminase has several isoenzyme forms, from muscle, heart and liver. It is important to identify the source of the isoenzyme before undertaking a long and exhaustive list of investigations. In Duchenne muscular dystrophy creatinine kinase and alanine transaminase are raised and abnormal from fetal life and before clinical symptoms are evident.

ANSWER 2.5

1. Hyperinflated right lung
   Tracheal and mediastinal shift to the left
   Low volume left lung
2. Visual inspection of chest
   Percussion

On inspection the right side of the chest was noted to be hyperinflated and moving less well than the left. Percussion note was more resonant on right. The combination suggests air trapping in all or part of the right lung. The appearances are strongly suggestive of a ball valve obstruction in a major airway on the right. The history suggests that this could well have been inhalation of a foreign body. At bronchoscopy a peanut was removed from the right main bronchus and the baby subsequently recovered uneventfully.

Paper 3 *Questions*

3

QUESTION 3.1

A male infant was born at 41 weeks' gestation, being the first child of healthy unrelated parents. His mother had a history of recreational drug usage (amphetamines and cannabis) during the first trimester. The membranes had ruptured 48 hours before delivery and his mother developed a pyrexia (38°C) during labour. For this reason he was commenced on intravenous penicillin and gentamicin after blood cultures had been taken. He initially fed well but at 9 hours of age was found to be having a generalised seizure which lasted approximately 10 minutes. Investigations were as follows:

Full blood count	normal
Serum electrolytes, calcium, magnesium	normal
Blood glucose	normal
Urine toxicology	negative
CSF microscopy	normal

A cranial ultrasound revealed generalised cerebral oedema with no other abnormalities, confirmed by CT scan. He continued to have generalised seizures despite appropriate doses of several anticonvulsants. Blood and CSF cultures were negative, as was PCR for herpes simplex virus. An EEG was performed (Fig. 3.1, p18):

1. What does the EEG show?
2. Suggest what occurred at the point marked on the EEG.

QUESTION 3.2

A 4-year-old girl presents to the orthopaedic surgeons with a swollen left knee 2 days after a fall in the school playground. On examination she is febrile (axillary temperature 38.7°C) and her knee is tender, swollen and red with limited painful movements. During the examination her mother says that she has had several boils on her back that have required incision and drainage.

Haemoglobin	10.8 g/dl
White cell count	$20.8 \times 10^9/l$

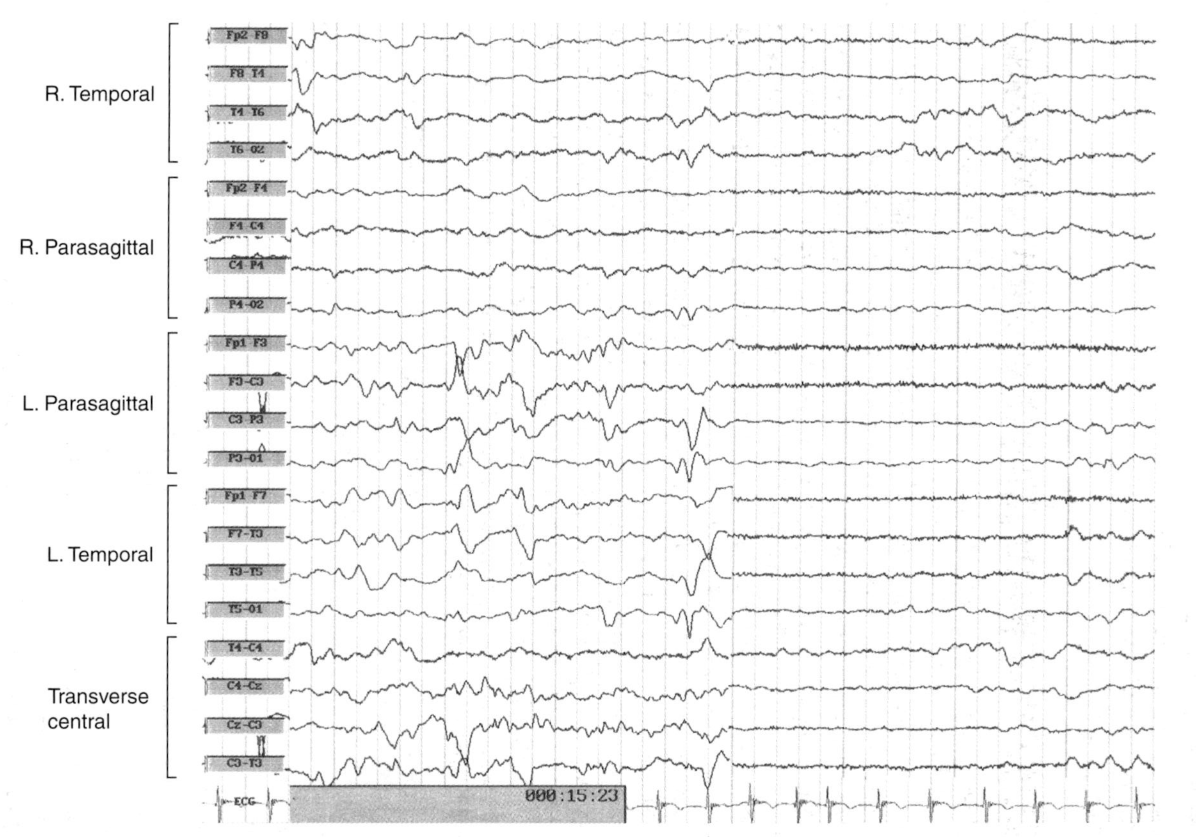
R. Temporal
R. Parasagittal
L. Parasagittal
L. Temporal
Transverse central
Fp2-F8
F8-T4
T4-T6
T6-O2
Fp2-F4
F4-C4
C4-P4
P4-O2
Fp1-F3
F3-C3
C3-P3
P3-O1
Fp1-F7
F7-T3
T3-T5
T5-O1
T4-C4
C4-Cz
Cz-C3
C3-T3
ECG
000:15:23

Fig. 3.1

Platelets	$201 \times 10^9/l$
ESR	84 mm/h
C-reactive protein	105 mg/l (normal < 5 mg/l)
Radiograph of the knee	normal

1. What is the diagnosis?
2. How can this be confirmed?
3. What is the underlying condition?
4. How is this inherited?

QUESTION 3.3

A 6-year-old girl presented with fever, lethargy and neck stiffness. Three days before she had been perfectly well. Her symptoms began with a coryzal illness and a non-productive cough. The next day she felt intermittently hot and cold with generalised muscle aches. The day before presentation she complained of a slightly sore neck, which became painful to move. She vomited after coughing on several occasions. Her general condition deteriorated on the day of admission. Her past medical history was unremarkable other than a head injury following a fall at the age of 18 months. She had recently returned from a family holiday in Thailand.

On examination she was well grown, normotensive, tachypnoeic, well hydrated, febrile and in considerable discomfort. Tripod and Kernig's signs were positive. There were no neurological signs and fundoscopy was normal. She had no photophobia. No rashes were seen. Examination of her abdomen, joints, ears, nose and throat were normal, as was her respiratory system, other than a slightly dull percussion note at the right apex. Assessment of her cardiovascular system was unremarkable. A CT scan of her head was normal. A lumbar puncture was then performed:

CSF microscopy	2 white blood cells/mm^3, 15 red blood cells/mm^3
Protein	0.2 g/l
Glucose	3.7 mmol/l
No organisms seen on Gram stain	

Haemoglobin	11.9 g/dl
White cell count	$14.6 \times 10^9/l$
Platelets	$298 \times 10^9/l$
ESR	87 mm/h
Prothrombin time	14 s (control 11–15 s)
Activated partial thromboplastin time	31 s (control 24–35 s)
Fibrinogen	3.5 g/l (normal 1.5–4.0 g/l)
Blood glucose	4.9 mmol/l

1. What is the likely cause for her neck stiffness?
2. How would you confirm the diagnosis?
3. What is the likely causative organism?

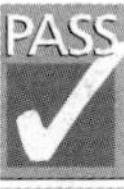

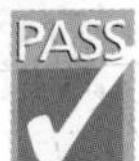

QUESTION 3.4

A 14-year-old boy presents complaining of shortness of breath, non-productive cough and lethargy. He is a known asthmatic and recently has been very well controlled on inhaled steroids. He is otherwise fit and well. He attended the Accident and Emergency department 1 month ago, having fallen from a horse, but was discharged home. He has eaten poorly but his mother is uncertain whether he has lost any weight. He has not been abroad or visited a farm recently. His 6-year-old sister has type 1 diabetes. The family have numerous pets including two dogs, a hamster and three budgies.

On examination, his temperature is 37.2°C and his oxygen saturation is 91% in air. He is dyspnoeic at rest with a respiratory rate of 32/min. He has neither finger clubbing nor lymphadenopathy. His chest wall movements are unequal and associated with mild subcostal recession. On percussion there is dullness on the left side anteriorly and posteriorly from the base to the mid zone. On auscultation, breath sounds are normal in all lung fields except the left mid zone and base, where they are difficult to hear. Palpation of his abdomen elicits mild tenderness in the epigastric region. There is no hepatospenomegaly and his testes are normal. His chest radiograph shows a pleural effusion which is tapped. The fluid shows the following:

Table 3.1

	Pleural fluid	*Serum*
Protein (g/l)	40	64
LDH (U/l)	301	132
Red blood cells/ml	100 000	
White blood cells/ml	1 000	

Cytology after cytospin — No abnormal cells seen

1. List five other investigations you would perform.
2. What are the most likely diagnoses? Give two.

QUESTION 3.5

A 2-year-old Omani boy presented with a 1-week history of high fever. His parents said that for 2–3 months before this he had not been eating well and had had abdominal distension and some vomiting. Until then he had been a well child. He had been born in Oman and the family moved to the UK when he was 18 months old. The rest of the family was well. They thought the child was growing normally and making normal developmental progress. His immunisation schedule was up to date. They thought he had been given his BCG at birth. He had had normal stools, no rash and no joint symptoms. There had been no abnormal bleeding or bruising.

On examination he was thin and pale with a temperature of 39°C. There was some cervical lymphadenopathy. His abdomen was distended and his spleen was palpable 4 cm below the left costal margin. There was no other organomegaly or lymphadenopathy, no petechiae or bruising, no rash and no joint abnormalities.

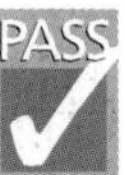

Haemoglobin	7.8 g/dl
MCV	56 fl
White cell count	$4.3 \times 10^9/l$
Platelets	$83 \times 10^9/l$
Urine culture	negative
Blood culture	negative
Chest radiograph	normal
Mantoux test	negative

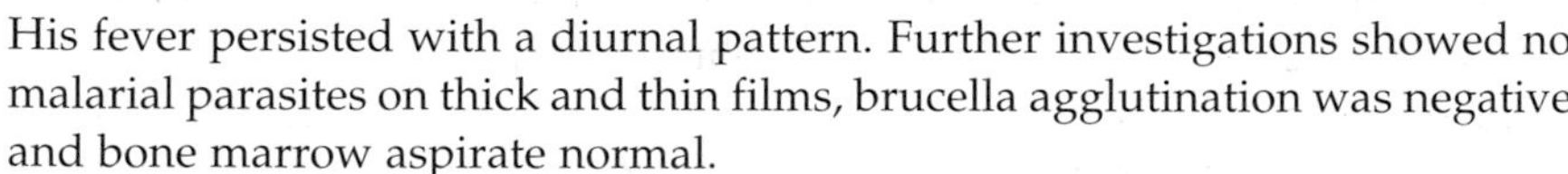
His fever persisted with a diurnal pattern. Further investigations showed no malarial parasites on thick and thin films, brucella agglutination was negative and bone marrow aspirate normal.

1. What is the most likely explanation for this child's illness?

Paper 3 *Answers*

3

ANSWER 3.1

1. Multifocal seizure discharges in both hemispheres, which are markedly reduced after the point marked
2. Administration of intravenous pyridoxine

Pyridoxine-dependent seizures are well recognised as a cause of intractable seizures in both neonates and infants. It is autosomal recessive, with a prevalence of at least 1:100 000. It is thought to be due to a defect in glutamic acid decarboxylase, although this is not as yet entirely proven. Patients classically exhibit seizures within hours of birth although some may have exhibited convulsive movements in utero. The presentation may be with a variety of seizure disorders, which, if severe, may result in a secondary encephalopathy. Although the seizures generally respond well to pyridoxine there are often developmental problems, especially affecting expressive language.

ANSWER 3.2

1. Staphylococcal septic arthritis of the left knee
2. Aspiration of the joint with culture of the synovial fluid
3. Chronic granulomatous disease
4. X-linked recessive in most instances; this case is one of the autosomal recessive cases

Chronic granulomatous disease (CGD) presents in most cases as recurrent staphylococcal skin abscesses. The CGD phenotype is the final consequence of one of several different molecular derangements that are inherited as either X-linked recessive or autosomal recessive; the former tends to be more severe than the latter. Five different biochemical defects in the oxidative chain of activated neutrophils have been described. Deficiency of a membrane receptor is autosomal recessive. The end result of all these defects, lack of the oxidative burst and production of reactive oxygen species, is uniform, as is the clinical manifestation. Neutrophils in CGD are unable to produce reactive oxygen species and therefore patients are susceptible to catalase-producing

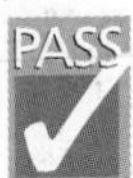

organisms (*Staphylococcus aureus, Aspergillus fumigatus, Klebsiella, Escherichia coli, Shigella, Salmonella, Pseudomonas*).

Management consists of aggressive antibiotic treatment of confirmed infections. Granulocyte transfusions may be of use in infections not responding to antibiotics. Steroids may be used to shrink some granulomata. Prophylactic antibiotics, interferon gamma and, in severe cases, bone marrow transplant are required.

ANSWER 3.3

1. Right upper lobe pneumonia
2. Chest radiography
3. *Streptococcus pneumoniae*

A negative lumbar puncture, the absence of photophobia or a rash combined with the presence of a fever, cough, tachypnoea and reduced air entry at the right apex make a right upper lobe pneumonia the most likely cause of this child's neck stiffness. Referred pain is well recognised with pneumonia. Lower lobe pneumonia can mimic an acute abdomen; upper lobe infection can cause neck stiffness.

ANSWER 3.4

1. Serum amylase
   Pleural fluid amylase
   Abdominal ultrasound
   CT scan of abdomen
   Magnetic resonance cholangiopancreatogram (MRCP)
2. Pancreatic trauma
   Low-grade pancreatitis

This boy presents with a pleural effusion after previous trauma. The pleural fluid analysis confirms a haemorrhagic exudate but with a relatively low white count. Causes of haemorrhagic effusions include trauma, pancreatic disease, malignancy, pulmonary embolism or a coagulopathy.

ANSWER 3.5

1. Visceral leishmaniasis

Unexplained fever in a child from Oman suggests the possibility of tropical disease. The pattern of fever is not typical of malaria and no parasites were identified. Brucellosis is common in communities where unpasteurised sheep or goat milk is consumed but the degree of splengomegaly is atypical and the cultures were negative. Splenomegaly of this degree with fever in a child from a desert country is strongly suggestive of visceral leishmaniasis (kala-azar). Infection occurs when female sandflies inject the promastigotes of *Leishmania dovanii* into the bloodstream, where they are engulfed by macrophages and replicate. Local replication results in cutaneous disease; dissemination leads to visceral disease. Dogs or other carnivores are usually the reservoir. The incubation period varies from a few weeks to 8 months. The onset is often abrupt in younger children and more insidious as they get older. Treatment is with stibogluconate or meglumine antimonate intravenously or intramuscularly.

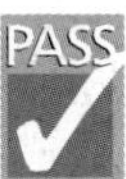

Paper 4 *Questions*

4

QUESTION 4.1

An 11-month-old boy was admitted with a 2-week history of chestiness and a 2-day history of lethargy. This had been preceded by a 6-week history of vomiting after meals. There was no overt difficulty with swallowing but this occasionally precipitated coughing. There had been no problems in pregnancy, delivery or the neonatal period. His parents had noticed that his cry had become quieter since the age of 5 months and he had stopped babbling since just before the onset of his chest problem. He had been able to roll onto his side from the age of 5 months but had not progressed further. His parents were unrelated. The only other history of note was that their first child had collapsed and died at the age of 20 hours with apparent hypoxic ischaemic encephalopathy.

On examination he was pale and listless. His weight was on the 10th centile and his head circumference on the 90th. His respiratory rate was 30/min, with good bilateral air entry. He was markedly hypotonic with increased limb reflexes, brisk palmar and plantar grasp reflexes and marked nystagmus on lateral gaze. Fundoscopy was normal.

1. Suggest a possible diagnosis.
2. List five investigations you would perform.

QUESTION 4.2

A female infant was born by emergency caesarean section at 33 weeks' gestation after her mother presented with a 4-day history of reduced fetal movements. This was the mother's second infant; her first was born by normal delivery 2 years ago. The infant weighed 1650 g and required intubation at birth for failure to sustain respiration. Her cord pH (arterial) was 7.34. She was transferred to the neonatal unit. She was easy to ventilate on low pressures and with no additional oxygen requirement. It was noted that she moved very little and did not 'fight the ventilator'. No paralysis or sedation was necessary.

Haemoglobin	13.4 g/dl
White cell count	18×10^9/ml
Platelets	17×10^9/ml

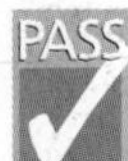

Cranial ultrasound scan:

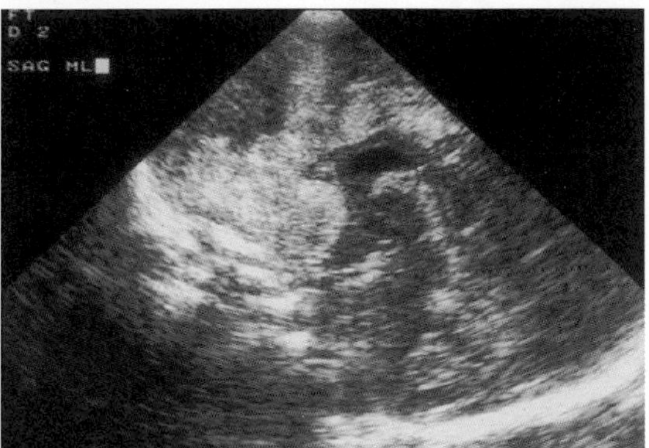

Fig. 4.1a

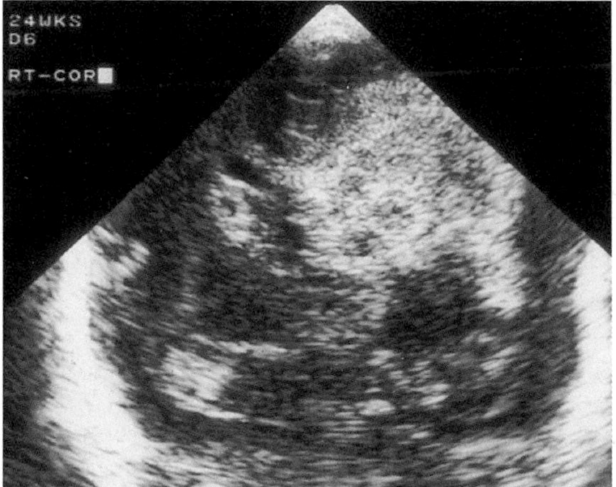

Fig. 4.1b

1. What does the scan show?
2. What is the underlying disorder?
3. What investigations would you like to perform?

QUESTION 4.3

A 15-year-old Afro-Caribbean girl presented with a 2-week history of pleuritic chest pain, nausea, abdominal cramps, lethargy and anorexia. She was reviewed and treated with oral erythromycin and dihydrocodeine. Her symptoms failed to improve and 3 days later she became febrile and complained of urinary frequency, urgency and dysuria. At the age of 13 years she had been diagnosed with polyarticular arthritis and had been treated with regular ibuprofen ever since.

On examination she was febrile with mild bilateral ankle oedema. Examination of her joints was unremarkable. Her blood pressure was 145/95 mmHg.

Urine dipstick	+++ blood, +++ protein
Urine microscopy	distorted red blood cells, mixed granular casts and scanty bacilli
Urine culture	no growth
Haemoglobin	8.4 g/dl
White cell count	4.2×10^9/l
Platelets	135×10^9/l
ESR	116 mm/h
C-reactive protein	34 mg/l (normal <5 mg/l)
Serum sodium	131 mmol/l
Serum potassium	5.9 mmol/l
Serum bicarbonate	16 mmol/l
Serum urea	33 mmol/l
Serum creatinine	445 μmol/l
Serum aspartate transaminase	28 IU/l (normal 10–45 IU/l)
Serum alkaline phosphatase	289 IU/l

1. What is the diagnosis?
2. List four investigations you would perform.
3. What is the usual treatment of this presentation?

QUESTION 4.4

A 9-year-old boy presents to the Accident and Emergency department shocked, having had a significant haematemesis. He becomes haemodynamically stable with a rapid infusion of 20 ml/kg of colloid. On examination, he is pale but alert. There is no finger clubbing or palmar erthyema. His weight is on the 25th centile and his height is on the 50th. There is no lymphadenopathy. Clinical examination is unremarkable, apart from splenomegaly of 7 cm and mild ascites. In the past he had a double-exchange transfusion in the neonatal period for ABO incompatibility and has been well since. There is no family history of note.

Haemoglobin	8.9 g/dl
White cell count	2.3×10^9/l
Neutrophils	1.2×10^9/l
Lymphocytes	1.0×10^9/l
Platelets	86×10^9/l
Reticulocyte count	2%
Blood film	normochromic, normocyctic, nil else
Coombs test	negative
Osmotic fragility test	negative
Serum albumin	39 g/l
Serum alanine transaminase	23 IU/l (normal 2–53 IU/l)
Serum bilirubin	14 μmol/l
Serum gamma glutamyl transferase	30 IU/l (normal 5–55 IU/l)
Prothrombin time	17 s (control 11–15 s)
Activated partial thromboplastin time	30 s (control 24–35 s)

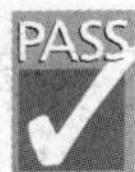

1. What is the diagnosis?
2. List four investigations that you would like to perform.
3. Name four steps in this child's management.

QUESTION 4.5

An 8-month-old baby presented with a 4-day history of loose stools and fever for a week. He had been born at 37 weeks, weighing 2775 g. The pregnancy and neonatal period had been uneventful apart from maternal constipation for which the mother was taking laxatives. He had initially been breast fed. Weaning had occurred uneventfully at 4 months and he was on mixed feeds with formula. He had always tended to vomit after feeds but this had improved with Gaviscon.

On examination his weight was 5.11 kg, length 69 cm, head circumference 42.5 cm and temperature 38.4°C. He was approximately 10% dehydrated and had marked muscle wasting. Blood pressure was 70 mmHg systolic. He was conscious and there were no other abnormal neurological signs.

Haemoglobin	15.1 g/dl
White cell count	22.5×10^9/l (lymphocytes 75%, neutrophils 18%)
Serum sodium	129 mmol/l
Serum potassium	1.9 mmol/l
Serum chloride	82 mmol/l
Serum creatinine	64 μmol/l
Serum urea	8.2 mmol/l
Serum pH	7.47
Base deficit	+3 mmol/l
Urinary sodium	5 mmol/l
Urinary potassium	20 mmol/l
Urinary urea	8.8 mmol/l

Following intravenous rehydration and potassium replacement he gained 160 g but continued to have a hypokalaemic alkalosis (serum potassium 2.2 mmol/l, pH 7.54, base deficit +5 mmol/l) even on 1.5 g KCl per day.

1. Suggest three possible diagnoses.
2. Give three relevant investigations.

Paper 4 *Answers*

4

ANSWER 4.1

1. Leigh's disease.
2. Blood lactate
   Blood pyruvate
   CSF lactate
   CSF pyruvate
   MRI brain scan

The diagnosis of Leigh's disease (subacute necrotising encephalomyelopathy) is suggested by the history of hypotonia, developmental regression and brainstem signs. This is a progressive neurodegenerative disorder with an onset in approximately 80% of cases in infancy, progressing to death within 2 years. Later onset disease and/or slower progression have been reported. Brainstem signs include respiratory problems, nystagmus and ophthalmoplegia. Other signs include ataxia, dystonia and optic atrophy. Defects of the pyruvate dehydrogenase complex (autosomal recessive), cytochrome oxidase and mitochondrial DNA have been documented in many patients. Deficiency of Complex I of the respiratory chain is also a recognised association and the gene mutation for Complex IV deficiency has recently been identified. Diagnosis is made by demonstrating the characteristic symmetrical lesions in the brainstem or basal ganglia (Fig. 4.2) along with a raised CSF lactate level.

ANSWER 4.2

1. (a) Subdural haematoma; (b) cerebral echogenicity consistent with intraventricular haemorrhage and haemorrhagic venous infarction
2. Neonatal alloimmune thrombocytopenia
3. Maternal IgG alloantibodies against a fetal platelet specific alloantigen, most commonly human platelet antigen 1a (HPA-1a)

Alloimmune thrombocytopenia is a serious fetal disorder resulting from platelet-antigen incompatibility between thc mother and fetus. HPA-1a is the most frequently involved, accounting for 80–90% of the cases. The diagnosis is usually made after the discovery of unexpected neonatal thrombocytopenia.

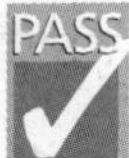

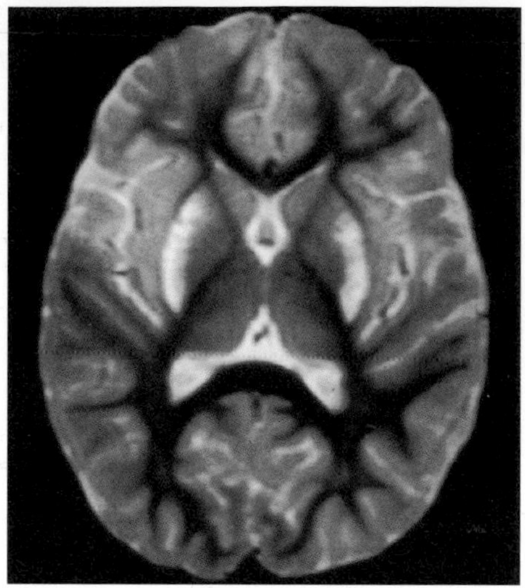

Fig. 4.2

Approximately 10–20% of affected fetuses have intracranial haemorrhages, one-quarter to one-half of which occur in utero. It is more severe in fetuses with an older affected sibling who had had an antenatal intracranial haemorrhage. Up to 20% of mothers do not have detectable antibodies; when they are present there is little correlation between levels and disease severity, making screening of mothers alone unreliable.

Future pregnancies are likely to be affected and therefore fetal blood sampling to determine fetal platelet phenotype should be undertaken at a gestation of about 20 weeks. Treatment begins when fetal thrombocytopenia is detected and includes maternal intravenous immunoglobulin, maternal steroids and in-utero platelet transfusions.

ANSWER 4.3

1. Systemic lupus erythematosus (SLE)
2. Renal biopsy
   C3, C4, C1q
   Double-stranded DNA
   Anti-nuclear antibody titre
3. Intravenous cyclophosphamide and oral prednisolone

This adolescent had SLE with lupus nephritis. Sickle-cell disease is a very unlikely diagnosis in this case, as she would have presented much earlier in life. Patients with sickle-cell trait do not present in this fashion and would be expected to have a higher haemoglobin. At diagnosis with SLE, renal involvement of varying degrees is seen in half to two-thirds of all children. Her renal lupus was severe with marked impairment of renal function, hypertension and heavy proteinuria. Her ankle oedema suggests she had nephrotic range proteinuria. Although not mentioned in the question her C3 and C4 were both depressed, a pattern frequently seen in renal lupus. A low C3 and low C4 can also be seen in membranoproliferative glomerulonephritis type I and rarely with systemic infection. A renal biopsy is often required in order to classify the severity of the nephritis. The nature of the nephritis determines the type of the treatment required. Currently, initial treatment of severe lupus nephritis is usually with pulsed intravenous cyclophosphamide in combination with oral steroids. Azathioprine is often given later as maintenance therapy. The renal prognosis is guarded.

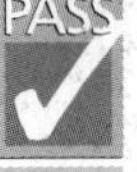

ANSWER 4.4

1. Portal vein thrombosis with secondary portal hypertension and hypersplenism
2. Abdominal ultrasound
   Endoscopy
   Angiography
   Thrombophilia screen
3. Oesphageal banding or sclerotherapy
   H_2 antagonist
   Avoidance of non-steroidal drugs and aspirin
   Vascular assessment for portocaval shunt

Portal venous thrombosis and associated cavernomatous formation will often present clinically with signs of portal hypertension, particularly haematemesis before the diagnosis is suspected. As this is an extrahepatic obstruction, with the development of collateral vessels around the malformation/thrombus, there is normal synthetic function of the liver. Splenomegaly is present and thus haemolytic disease needs to be excluded. Ascites is usually present only after a large gastrointestinal bleed. The aetiology is diagnosed radiologically and is also important in assessing for corrective surgery. Over 50% of children do not have a history of neonatal sepsis, dehydration or umbilical vein catheterisation.

ANSWER 4.5

1. Bartter's syndrome
   Gitelman's syndrome
   Laxative abuse
2. Serum aldosterone
   Serum renin
   Serum magnesium

A persistent hypokalaemia with a metabolic alkalosis of this degree is typical of Bartter's syndrome, of which three subtypes are described: type I: Serum Na^+K^+-2 cotransporter; type II: K^+ channel; III: Cl^- channel defects, all of

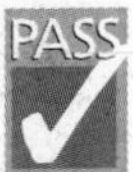

which result in intravascular volume reduction and a rise in hyperaldosterone and renin levels. The blood pressure is usually normal. The disorder is prostaglandin mediated and can be treated with COX-1 or possibly COX-2 inhibitors. The differential diagnosis includes Gitelman's syndrome (as Bartter's but usually with hypomagnesaemia), familial hypokalaemic alkalosis with tubulopathy, prolonged diuretic use and extrarenal chloride loss (laxative abuse, chloridorrhoea, cystic fibrosis). This child had no history of diarrhoea or diuretic use. The maternal laxative therapy was probably incidental. His serum magnesium was normal. Aldosterone and renin levels were both raised. Treatment with indomethacin resulted in normal potassium levels and acid–base balance without potassium supplements.

Paper 5 *Questions*

5

QUESTION 5.1

A 12-year-old boy was referred with a 4-week history of lethargy, unsteadiness, limb and abdominal pain and constipation. In the preceding few days he had also become aggressive. His school work was said to have deteriorated markedly since the onset of his symptoms. On examination his blood pressure was 140/90 mmHg, he had facial weakness, areflexia, ataxia and was unable to feel objects in his hand.

1. Suggest a possible diagnosis
2. What investigations would you perform? (List three.)
3. List three ways in which you would manage the condition.

QUESTION 5.2

An 18-year-old mother with pregnancy-induced hypertension gave birth by Caesarean section to a premature male infant weighing 1305 g at 32 weeks' gestation. Apgar scores were 6 at 1 min and 8 at 5 min. During the first postnatal week, he required surfactant and ventilation for respiratory distress syndrome, and phototherapy for hyperbilirubinaemia, but he did well and his condition stabilised. Cranial ultrasound scan at this time was normal.

Two weeks postnatally he was re-intubated for respiratory failure secondary to sepsis. He developed a rash, presumed candidal in origin, which was treated with topical clotrimazole. He also received antibiotics and amphotericin in view of suspected bacterial and/or fungal sepsis. All blood cultures were negative.

Three and a half weeks postnatally, he had an episode of gross haematuria with evidence of acute renal failure. Examination of the abdomen revealed a large tender mass in the left flank region. Ultrasound of this showed a swollen enlarged kidney that was echogenic with prominent medullary pyramids. A cranial ultrasound examination performed at the same time showed echodensities in the germinal matrix bilaterally. Two days later there was a progressive neurological deterioration with lethargy leading to coma. A cranial ultrasound was repeated. This showed bilateral echodensities in the periventricular white matter, germinal matrix, thalamus, and ventricle.

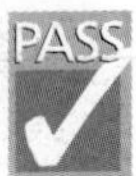

Despite treatment of the renal failure, the baby died 31 days after birth, without any improvement in neurological status.

1. Give three reasons why this infant's renal function might have deteriorated.
2. What two further investigations would you perform to exclude fungal sepsis?
3. What is the connection between the renal pathology and the final cranial ultrasound appearance?
4. What conditions would you want to exclude?

QUESTION 5.3

A 4-year-old boy with short bowel syndrome attended with abdominal pain. His pain started 3 weeks before his presentation. It was intermittent, lasting for about 20 minutes at a time and severe enough to cause the boy to cry. It occurred about three times a day and was located in the right loin. He was sometimes woken from sleep by the pain. There were no obvious exacerbating or relieving factors. The frequency had not changed with time.

He was born at 27 weeks' gestation, weighing 1100 g. He had a stormy neonatal course, suffering from severe necrotising enterocolitis. Ultimately he had an extensive resection of his ileum. Despite a number of gastrointestinal complications he was eventually discharged home on enteral nasogastric feeds. Following an intensive behavioural feeding programme he took much of his nutrition by mouth. He was particularly keen on strawberries although they often led to looser stools.

In the past he had had several hospital admissions with upper respiratory tract infections. These led to respiratory compromise because of his chronic lung disease. He was known to have mild global developmental delay.

On examination, his weight was on the 0.4th centile and his height on the 3rd centile. He was bright and alert, afebrile, well hydrated and not icteric. During an episode of pain he had tenderness in his upper abdomen and right flank, although assessment was difficult. Bowel sounds were heard.

Urine dipstick	+++ blood, trace protein
Urine microscopy	numerous red blood cells, many crystals
Urine culture	no growth

1. Suggest five possible diagnoses, in order of likelihood.
2. Give six further pertinent investigations.

QUESTION 5.4

A 13-year-old girl presents with an 8-week history of pain in her right knee and difficulty in weight bearing. Though she is a keen gymnast, there has been no history of trauma. She now complains of a severe constant burning pain in her lower leg and cannot tolerate having her trousers on because of the pain. There is no history of difficulty in micturition or defaecation. As a 3-year-old girl she was admitted to hospital with an irritable hip that resolved with conservative treatment, otherwise past medical history is unremarkable. She has no siblings. Her maternal grandmother has rheumatoid arthritis.

On examination, she is afebrile and normotensive. She will not weight bear on her right leg. Her right calf appears wasted. She complains of severe pain with gentle touching both above and below her knee anteriorly. The range of movement of her knee is restricted because of pain. The medial side of her calf is oedmatous and cool to touch. All peripheral pulses are palpable. Her ankle reflexes are present bilaterally and plantar reflexes are flexor.

Haemoglobin	13.0 g/dl
White cell count	$6.3 \times 10^9/l$
Platelets	$176 \times 10^9/l$
ESR	2 mm/h
Rheumatoid factor	negative
Autoantibody screen	negative
Urinalysis	negative
Radiograph knee	diffuse osteopenia around knee

1. What is the diagnosis?
2. What is the management?

QUESTION 5.5

A 3-year-old girl was admitted with a 6-day history of chickenpox and an 8-hour history of pain and stiffness in her arms. She had not been particularly unwell with the chickenpox. On the morning of admission she was eating breakfast when her hands went 'stiff and funny'. Her parents demonstrated a posture with flexure of the wrists and extension of the fingers. At the same time the left pupil appeared small and the eyelid droopy compared with the right. Her parents also noted that she appeared to be unsteady on her feet with a tendency to stagger to one side. She had been born at term, weighing 3790 g. The neonatal period had been uneventful and she had been making normal developmental progress to date. There was no significant family history.

On examination she was apyrexial and not ill. There were no dysmorphic features. Her height was on the 25th centile and her weight on the 10th. There were numerous chickenpox scabs in various stages of healing. There was some truncal ataxia with a tendency to veer to the right. Examination was unremarkable otherwise.

Haemoglobin	13 g/dl
White cell count	$7.3 \times 10^9/l$
Platelets	$130 \times 10^9/l$
Serum sodium	134 mmol/l
Serum potassium	3.9 mmol/l
Serum chloride	97 mmol/l
Serum calcium	1.14 mmol/l
Ionised calcium	0.5 mmol/l
Serum phosphate	2.48 mmol/l

Serum albumin	39 g/l
Serum magnesium	0.62 mmol/l

1. What is your provisional diagnosis?
2. What other six investigations would you carry out?

Paper 5 *Answers*

5

ANSWER 5.1

1. Heavy metal poisoning
2. Determination of possible exposure (from further history)
   Serum concentrations
   Environmental screening
3. Chelation therapy with monitoring of excretion
   Treat hypertension
   Remove source of environmental exposure

The diagnosis of heavy metal poisoning is suggested by the change in the boy's behaviour and deteriorating school work along with a peripheral neuropathy. The presence of the latter makes a space-occupying lesion unlikely. Further questioning excluded lead exposure (the family home was modern with no lead piping or paint) but the patient had dismantled a barometer in his bedroom and had subsequently tried to dispose of the mercury using a vacuum cleaner, which may have dispersed the mercury further.

ANSWER 5.2

1. Renal venous thrombosis
   Obstructive uropathy secondary to fungal masses
   Renal toxicity of amphotericin
2. Urine microscopy from suprapubic aspiration sample
   Examination of retina for fungal masses
3. Hypercoagulable state leading to venous thromboses in both the kidneys and the cerebral venous sinuses
4. Factor V mutation (FV Leiden)
   Protein C deficiency
   Protein S deficiency

This ill neonate became dehydrated in a situation where the renal function was already at risk from fungal sepsis and from treatment with amphotericin. This precipitated a hypercoagulable state leading to widespread venous thromboses. These became clinically evident as renal venous thrombosis and later cerebral venous sinus thromboses.

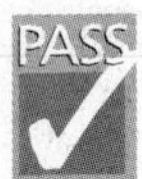

In paediatric practice, 90% of renal vein thrombosis occurs in infants less than 1 year old and 75% occur in infants under 1 month old. In infants, important factors associated with primary thrombosis of the internal cerebral or renal veins include diarrhoea, vomiting, and dehydration. Any factors causing increased coagulability of the blood may also contribute. Rarer, but important, causes include infants of diabetic mothers, factor V mutation, protein C and protein S deficiencies, antiphopholipid antibodies and systemic lupus. They may be seen with saphenous central venous lines.

Venous thrombosis is a clinically under-recognised cause of coma and seizures in the neonatal period. The dural venous sinuses are most commonly affected. In some cases, neonatal cerebral venous thrombosis may have a favourable outcome with normal subsequent neurodevelopment, although a poor outcome is more likely when the internal venous system is involved. The presence of haemorrhagic venous infarcts bilaterally in the deep hemispheres is characteristic of thrombosis of the internal cerebral venous system. Thrombosis of the internal cerebral venous system should be considered in the differential diagnosis of neonatal intraventricular haemorrhage and periventricular leukomalacia, particularly when the infant is near term and has bilateral haemorrhagic lesions.

ANSWER 5.3

1. Calcium oxalate renal stones
   Gallstones
   Bowel bacterial overgrowth
   Intestinal stricture
   Pseudo-obstruction
2. Urinary oxalate/creatinine ratio
   Ultrasound scan of renal tract/abdomen
   Abdominal radiograph
   Dietary assessment
   H_2 breath test
   Contrast study

The clinical picture is one of right renal colic. Hyperoxaluria is a well described complication of short bowel syndrome and can lead to calcium oxalate stone formation. In health, luminal calcium combines with dietary oxalate to form calcium oxalate, which is non-absorbable. Oxalate absorption from the colon is increased in this syndrome as excess non-absorbed fat binds luminal calcium to form soaps. The remaining soluble oxalate is readily absorbed. This child was consuming large quantities of strawberries, which are rich in oxalate. Treatment of hyperoxaluria is with a low oxalate diet. The other possible diagnoses produce pain that does not have the character or location of renal colic. Gallstones can be seen in short bowel syndrome. Malabsorption of bile acids as a consequence of ileal resection and bacterial colonisation leads to an increased incidence of biliary cholesterol stones. Bowel bacterial overgrowth can occasionally produce vague abdominal pain and is treated with broad-spectrum antibiotics. Pseudo-obstruction and intestinal stricture are also recognised problems in short bowel syndrome and are treated with prokinetic agents and surgery respectively.

ANSWER 5.4

1. Reflex sympathetic dystrophy
2. Intensive physiotherapy
   Analgesia
   Psychological assessment and support
   Consideration for a regional guanethidine block

Reflex sympathetic dystrophy is a clinical diagnosis. The children present with neuropathic pain and physical signs of autonomic dysfunction. The neuropathic pain includes burning, paraesthesia, dysaesthesia and pain provoked by a stimulus that would not normally cause pain. Autonomic changes include temperature changes, sweating, mottling and oedema. A history of trauma may be absent in over 50% of patients. The prognosis is better than in adults and centres on supportive management with intensive physiotherapy and pain control.

ANSWER 5.5

1. Hypoparathyroidism
2. Serum parathormone levels
   Slit-lamp examination of eyes
   Thyroid function
   T-cell numbers
   Autoantibody screen
   Chromosome analysis

The parathormone level in this girl was recorded at 0.4 IU/l (normal >10 IU/l). Other investigations were normal. Her serum calcium levels normalised on supplementary 1-α-cholecalciferol and she grew normally with no recurrence of symptoms. Hypoparathyroidism may occur in association with other abnormalities (CHARGE, VACTERL), or in association with microdeletions in the region of chromosome 22 (for example di George syndrome). An autosomal dominant form also occurs. A genetic basis has also been described in patients with hypoparathyroidism associated with other endocrine abnormalities (polyglandular endocrinopathy type 1) and with renal dysfunction, hypopituitarism and deafness. This girl's symptoms appeared after an intercurrent illness which makes an autoimmune basis more likely. Ataxia following chickenpox is commoner in children under 5 years of age and usually resolves spontaneously.

Paper 6 *Questions*

6

QUESTION 6.1

A 7-year-old boy presents with progressive weakness of all four limbs. He had previously been well, apart from a non-specific viral illness in the preceding week. For the previous 24 hours he had been lying immobile on the sofa at home, and was able to drink but not feed himself. His father wondered whether his breathing had been shallow. On examination he is appropriately grown, fully conscious, alert and taking interest in his surroundings. His limb tone is severely reduced, he is unable to stand or sit unsupported. He is able to reach out for toys but is unable to lift them. His muscles are generally tender. Peripheral reflexes are present and slightly increased in all four limbs. Plantar reflexes are extensor. He is pink in air with equal air entry; his respiratory rate is 35/min. The rest of the examination is normal.

1. Suggest two possible diagnoses.
2. Suggest three investigations.

QUESTION 6.2

A 3-week-old male infant has become lethargic, feeds poorly and has difficulty swallowing. His birthweight was 1325 g and he now weighs 1420 g. He has been bottle fed since birth. There has been no vomiting and no diarrhoea. He was born by normal vaginal delivery at 34^{+4} weeks' gestation and admitted to the neonatal unit. He was started on preterm formula milk in view of the intrauterine growth retardation. He is afebrile and the rest of the examination is unremarkable apart from mild jaundice. His GP telephones shortly after his admission to say that his Guthrie test is positive.

Full blood count	normal
Serum urea and electrolytes	normal
Urine culture	negative
Blood cultures	negative
Serum amino acid profile	elevated levels of tyrosine and phenylalanine

1. What is the likely diagnosis?
2. What is the treatment?
3. What is the eventual prognosis?

QUESTION 6.3

A 9-year-old girl was reviewed 3 months after a successful cadaveric renal transplant, and had a temperature of 40.5°C. She felt generally unwell and on examination was noted to have significant tonsillar enlargement without exudates and marked bilateral cervical lymphadenopathy. Her transplanted kidney was non-tender.

She originally presented with chronic renal failure secondary to severe reflux nephropathy and was transplanted before requiring dialysis. At the time of transplantation all serological tests for cytomegalovirus (CMV) and Epstein–Barr virus (EBV) proved negative. The donor was a 10-year-old road traffic accident victim who was also CMV negative. The operation was uncomplicated and she made a good initial postoperative recovery. Standard immunosuppression with cyclosporin A, azathioprine and prednisolone was used. At 8 days post-transplant she developed steroid-resistant acute cellular rejection which was treated with anti-thymocyte globulin. Her renal function returned to baseline and no further rejection episodes were encountered.

Serum sodium	144 mmol/l
Serum potassium	4.9 mmol/l
Serum urea	7.8 mmol/l
Serum creatinine	118 μmol/l (87 mmol/l the previous week)
Serum aspartate transaminase	14 IU/l (normal 10–45 IU/l)
Serum alanine transaminase	4 IU/l (normal 0–25 IU/l)
Ultrasound scan of transplanted kidney	normal
Urine microscopy	scanty red blood cells only
CMV PCR	negative
EBV PCR	positive

1. Give two possible diagnoses.
2. Suggest four further investigations.

QUESTION 6.4

A 4-month-old infant brought into casualty in a semi-conscious state is floppy, and responds poorly to painful stimuli. He is afebrile, jaundiced and looks approximately 5–10% dehydrated. On examination he is not maintaining his airway by himself and his respiratory rate is 80/min with a shallow respiratory pattern. His oxygen saturation in air is 90%. His pulse rate is 160/min, and capillary refill is 4 seconds. His heart sounds are normal with thready peripheral pulses palpable. On abdominal examination, he has a firm liver 4 cm palpable below the costal margin and a palpable spleen tip. He has normal genitalia. His anterior fontanelle is flat and fundoscopy is normal.

He was born at term to consanguineous parents. He has been exclusively breast fed from birth and has thrived. He is not yet weaned. Recently he has been sufficiently disturbed by colic for his mother to give him anti-colic medication. Over the last 72 hours he has become more lethargic, with progressive vomiting that is now projectile. His mother is uncertain of when he had his last wet nappy. In the family history, his elder brother had pyloric stenosis and his sister was born with talipes.

Haemoglobin	11.0 g/dl
White cell count	7.8×10^9/l
Platelets	93×10^9/l
Prothrombin time	23 s (control 11–15 s)
Activated partial thromboplastin time	49 s (control 24–35 s)
Blood glucose	1.9 mmol/l
Capillary pH	7.11
Base deficit	–9.6 mmol/l
Total protein	67 g/l
Serum albumin	35 g/l
Serum bilirubin	77 μmol/l
Alanine tramsaminase	1666 IU/l (normal 2–53 IU/l)
Aspartate transaminase	1301 IU/l (normal 10–45 IU/l)
Gamma glutamyl transferase	323 IU/l (normal 5–55 IU/l)
Urine microscopy	negative
Urinalysis	++ protein
Urinary succinyl acetone	not detected

1. What further investigations would you undertake? (List five.)
2. What is the diagnosis?

QUESTION 6.5

A baby girl weighing 3500 g was born at term to healthy unrelated parents. She needed no resuscitation and went to the postnatal ward with her mother. Breast feeding was successfully established. At the discharge examination on day 4 the baby was noted to have stridor, which was worse when she became agitated. The mother said that the stridor had been present since birth but had become more noticeable. In addition she commented that the baby sounded as if it had a sore throat. Otherwise the baby was well but feeding had latterly become more difficult because she appeared to need pauses to get her breath.

Examination revealed a well baby who was pink and well perfused in air. There was noticeable inspiratory and expiratory stridor at rest, which became worse when the baby was disturbed. The respiratory rate was 40/min, there was minimal subcostal recession but an obvious tracheal tug. Air entry was equal and normal. The cry was a little hoarse. Examination was otherwise unremarkable.

1. Give three possible reasons for the clinical signs.
2. Suggest three investigations that might help elucidate the cause.

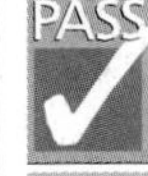

Paper 6 *Answers*

6

ANSWER 6.1

1. Transverse myelitis
   Acute disseminated encephalomyelitis (ADEM)
2. MRI brain/spinal cord
   Serum serology
   CSF serology

There are a number of features that might suggest Guillain–Barré syndrome (shallow respiration, myalgia, reduced tone) but the preserved reflexes are not typical of a demyelinating peripheral neuropathy. Transverse myelitis often follows a non-specific viral infection, although some cases are related to *Mycoplasma* and *Borrelia* infection. Pain in the limbs and/or back is a common first symptom and the onset of severe weakness may occur rapidly. The discriminating features are a mixed pattern of upper and lower motor neurone signs. CSF examination commonly shows an increase in protein level, although it may be normal; the cell count is often raised. Imaging will reveal swelling of the cord and will exclude other lesions (for example tumours) compressing the cord. Treatment is supportive and analgesia is given for pain. There is no evidence that the prognosis is improved by the use of steroids or ACTH.

A similar presenting picture can result from ADEM, which results in patchy demyelination throughout the brain and spinal cord on MRI. The prognosis for both conditions is surprisingly good in childhood, with about 80% making a full recovery.

ANSWER 6.2

1. Transient tyrosinaemia of the newborn
2. Reduction of protein content of feeds to 2–3 g/kg/day (some advocate switching to breast feeds) Vitamin C 200–400 mg/day
3. Good, resolves spontaneously during the first month of life although some patients may have mild intellectual deficits

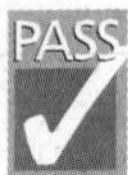

Transient tyrosinemia of the newborn is characterised by the transient build-up of tyrosine and phenylalanine in the blood. It affects 0.5–10% of newborn infants during the first 2–4 weeks of life. Preterm infants, and term infants on a high-protein diet are at risk. It is suggested that there is a delayed maturation of *p*-hydroxyphenyl-pyruvic acid oxidase that catalyses the conversion of tyrosine to *p*-OH-phenylpyruvic acid and most infants come to medical attention because of a positive Guthrie test. Management revolves around reduction of dietary protein to 2–3 g/kg/day (breast milk is ideal for this). Vitamin C (200–400 mg/day) may help optimal functioning of the enzyme. Overall the prognosis is good, with spontaneous resolution during the first month of life; some patients may eventually have mild intellectual deficits and decreased psycholinguistic abilities.

ANSWER 6.3

1. Acute renal rejection secondary to infectious mononucleosis
   Post-transplant lymphoproliferative disorder (PTLD)
2. Renal biopsy
   Chest radiograph
   Lymph node or tonsil biopsy
   Bone marrow aspirate

Although this child may have developed an acute EBV infection that has precipitated a second episode of rejection (which could be confirmed on renal biopsy), there are a number of features pointing to an alternative diagnosis of PTLD.

PTLD is an abnormal proliferation of lymphocytes occurring in the immunocompromised host after organ or bone marrow transplantation. The following applies specifically to PTLD following childhood renal transplantation. Its prevalence is 1–3% and the disease has a wide histopathological spectrum, ranging from a mild infectious mononucleosis-like illness to a monomorphic proliferation of lymphocytes similar to non-Hodgkin lymphoma. It is almost always associated with EBV infection and most often occurs in the first 3 months after renal transplantation, particularly if heavy immunosuppression was required. Common features include unexplained fever, tonsillar and adenoidal enlargement, superficial neck, mediastinal or mesenteric adenopathy, graft dysfunction and liver or spleen involvement. The diagnosis is usually made on a combination of biopsy (e.g. lymph node, tonsil) histopathology, immunophenotype and molecular studies. First-line treatment is by reducing immunosuppression and starting IV antiviral therapy with ganciclovir or acyclovir. The prognosis is usually good.

ANSWER 6.4

1. Urinary reducing substances
   Urinary tubular reabsorption of phosphate
   Urinary aminoacid screen
   Review of products in the anti-colic medication

Measurement of aldolase B activity in liver or intestinal mucosa when recovered
2. Hereditary fructose intolerance

Hereditary fructose intolerance, an autosomal recessive disorder, is due to fructose-1-phosphate deficiency. It presents following the introduction of sucrose- or fructose-containing foods or medication. Acutely, the infant will present with a history of significant vomiting, hepatomegaly and liver dysfunction. Initial treatment is supportive, with the removal of fructose, sucrose and sorbital from the diet, which must be maintained lifelong. The proteinuria reflects the associated Fanconi syndrome. Fanconi syndrome can have many aetiologies, including metabolic causes such as galactosaemia, cystinosis, tyrosinaemia and Wilson's disease.

ANSWER 6.5

1. Vocal cord palsy
   Mass or other obstructive lesion in larynx (e.g. cyst, tumour, web)
   Mass in superior mediastinum (e.g. lymphangioma, neuroblastoma)
2. Chest radiograph to visualise tracheal position
   Direct laryngoscopy
   CT imaging

The baby presents with very specific signs. The presence of inspiratory and expiratory stridor suggests that this is upper airway obstruction which is fixed and relatively severe. It is therefore very unlikely that this is laryngomalacia (which may be severe but never causes expiratory obstruction) or tracheomalacia associated with an aberrant vessel or fistula. The association with the hoarse cry makes it likely that the lesion is affecting one or both vocal cords. The baby had not been intubated at birth so direct trauma was unlikely, but this could have been an 'idiopathic' congenital cord palsy or resulting from a mass effect. The most common superior mediastinal masses arise from lymphohaemangiomata (cystic hygroma), goitres or neuroblastoma. Direct laryngoscopy revealed a large cyst on the left aryepiglottic fold. Diagnostic aspiration abolished the symptoms (the cyst fluid was transudate) but they recurred 2 weeks later, following which laser ablation was performed with a satisfactory result.

Paper 7 *Questions*

7

QUESTION 7.1

A set of twins (one male, one female) was delivered by Caesarean section at 33 weeks' gestation because of concerns regarding intrauterine growth retardation and deterioration in fetal biophysical profiles. They required minimal resuscitation at birth and had birthweights of 1150 g and 1000 g respectively. Their initial postnatal progress was satisfactory, they needed no respiratory support and were both started on enteral feeds on the second day of life. On day 5 both developed signs consistent with sepsis and both required ventilation. Blood and CSF cultures subsequently grew *Klebsiella* sp., which was also isolated from maternal milk. The female twin died as a result of overwhelming sepsis, despite appropriate antibiotic cover and the use of intravenous immunoglobulin and granulocyte colony-stimulating factor.

The surviving twin made a slow recovery from his infection and took several weeks to become fully re-established on enteral feeds, requiring parenteral nutrition in the interim. He became jaundiced and developed raised liver enzymes with hepatomegaly in association with his septicaemia; he remained jaundiced with mild hepatomegaly after his recovery, although he was otherwise well. He fed voraciously (8 fluid ounces every 2–3 hours), to such an extent that he was felt to have gastro-oesophageal reflux resulting in cough with desaturation. This responded in part to feed thickeners. His weight remained below but parallel to the third centile.

Full blood count and differential	normal
Serum immunoglobulins	normal
Serum bilirubin	235 μmol/l (90% conjugated)
Albumin	32 g/l (normal 30–45 g/l)
Alanine transferase	57 IU/l (normal 3–50 IU/l)
Alkaline phosphatase	693 IU/l (normal 150–375 IU/l)
Thyroid function	normal
Clotting screen	normal
HIDA scan	normal
Liver ultrasound	normal

1. Suggest two possible diagnoses.
2. List four investigations that you would perform?

QUESTION 7.2

A developmentally normal 4-year-old girl has been generally off colour for 3 weeks. She has lost weight and her appetite is poor. She developed a cough that did not respond to amoxicillin from her GP. After completion of the course she was referred for a chest radiograph. This showed a right upper lobe consolidation and she was admitted to hospital for intravenous antibiotics. On admission she was febrile and examination of her chest was in keeping with the radiological picture.

Haemoglobin	7.9 g/dl
White cell count	$10.3 \times 10^9/l$
Platelets	$333 \times 10^9/l$
Sputum culture	*Streptococcus pneumoniae* (sensitive to penicillin)

After 2 days of intravenous antibiotics she was clinically improving. She was discharged home on the third day to complete the course at home. Before discharge her mother mentioned that she did not appear to be walking as much as normal. Examination of her legs revealed no abnormalities, either of the joints or of the nervous system. Two weeks after discharge she was re-admitted by her GP with weakness of both legs and inability to stand. Examination revealed weakness of all muscle groups in her lower limbs, her reflexes were slightly brisk and plantars were flexor. She would not co-operate with testing sensation.

1. What is the likely cause of her weakness?
2. How do the two admissions relate to each other?
3. What urgent investigation would you perform?
4. What is the probable underlying diagnosis?

QUESTION 7.3

A 7-year-old boy presented to his GP with restlessness, difficulty in concentrating, poor sleeping and a poor appetite. A diagnosis of attention deficit hyperactivity disorder (ADHD) was made and methylphenidate commenced. The child had a history of eczema and wheezing. His mother suffered from depression and his father had type 1 diabetes mellitus.

Over the next few weeks the boy's symptoms worsened. He became increasingly restless and irritable, his insomnia worsened, his weight began to fall and he developed headaches and dizziness. He was then referred to the Accident and Emergency department. On examination he was thin, fidgety and difficult to engage. He had a fine tremor, his heart rate was regular at 140 beats/min and his systolic blood pressure was 130 mmHg.

1. Give two possible diagnoses.
2. Suggest investigations that would differentiate between these diagnoses.

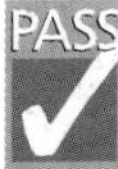

QUESTION 7.4

A 28-month-old boy is seen in outpatients as his parents have been concerned about the number of colds and ear infections that he has had. They describe him as always being 'snuffly' with a constant moist cough. He was admitted to hospital at 9 months of age with a right upper lobe pneumonia, which responded to intravenous antibiotics. He is the first child, born at term to non-consanguineous parents. He is fully immunised. He is described as clumsy and falls over easily, though he only started to walk at 16 months. On examination, he is a quiet placid infant. His weight is on the 25th centile and his height is on the 3rd centile. He is not dysmorphic. On auscultation to his chest there are fine crepitations at the left base.

Haemoglobin	11.2 g/l
White cell count	7.4×10^9/l
Neutrophils	5.2×10^9/l
Lymphocytes	1.1×10^9/l
Platelets	263×10^9/l
IgG	10.2 g/l (normal 3.0–11.0 g/l)
IgA	0.1 g/l (normal 0.3–1.4 g/l)
IgM	1.9 g/l (normal 0.5–2.0 g/l)
IgE	5 KU/l (20–125 KU/l)
Pneumococcal antibody titres	low
Tetanus antibody titres	low
Haemophilus antibody titres	low

1. What further six investigations would you carry out?
2. What is the diagnosis?

QUESTION 7.5

A 2-day-old term baby weighing 2940 g was referred to a local neonatal intensive care unit with recurrent apnoea and a distended abdomen. The apnoeic episodes were prolonged and severe and several had been treated with mask ventilation. Between them the baby appeared well and fed normally. Delivery had been by ventouse for a persistent high head but the baby breathed spontaneously within 4 minutes of birth. Cord arterial pH was 7.21 and Apgar scores were 5 at 1 minute and 8 at 5 minutes.

Clinical examination on admission revealed a normal-looking male infant with a moderately distended abdomen. Tone was generally reduced but there was no muscle wasting or fibrillation and tendon reflexes were normal. An abdominal radiograph showed diffuse dilatation of small and large bowel with gas, except for the rectum, which was empty. Over the 12 hours following admission the baby had three profound episodes of hypoventilation, the last of which resulted in the need for mechanical ventilation. It was noted that the episodes of hypoventilation were more likely to occur when he went to sleep. Investigations for infection were negative. Blood sugar, electrolytes and ammonia were normal.

1. Give two possible diagnoses.
2. Suggest treatment (if appropriate).

Paper 7 *Answers*

7

ANSWER 7.1

1. Cystic fibrosis
   Alpha-1-antitrypsin deficiency
2. Sweat test
   DNA probes for common cystic fibrosis mutations
   Stool elastase
   Alpha-1-antitrypsin phenotype

Cystic fibrosis is relatively rare as a cause of neonatal cholestasis (0.6–0.7% of cases) but must be excluded as a cause, especially in Caucasian infants. A proportion of cases will have respiratory symptoms and/or failure to thrive at presentation. Their prognosis with regard to their liver disease is good in the short to medium term. Clearly α-1-antitrypsin deficiency may also present in a similar fashion. Nutritional support using medium-chain triglyceride-based formula and fat-soluble vitamin supplementation is paramount in the management of patients with cholestatic jaundice.

ANSWER 7.2

1. Spinal cord compression
   Reject: Guillain–Barré or other causes of peripheral neuropathy
2. Growth of tumour causing cord compression and infiltration/obstruction of the right upper bronchus/lobe
3. Spinal cord MRI or CT
4. Neuroblastoma

This girl presents with an upper motor neurone weakness affecting her lower limbs only. Although Guillain–Barré may be considered, the distinguishing feature is the presence of reflexes (these are markedly diminished or absent in Guillain–Barré, which is a lower motor neurone disease). The absence of trauma and of pain with a non-specific history of ill health suggest neoplastic infiltration causing spinal cord compression. The involvement of spine and the chest symptoms/signs make neuroblastoma the most likely diagnosis in this age group. Treatment will depend on the staging of the disease and the results of genetic markers.

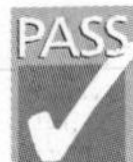

ANSWER 7.3

1. Methylphenidate hydrochloride toxicity
   Hyperthyroidism
2. T_4, T_3, TSH
   Plasma methylphenidate hydrochloride assay

This case is consistent with the diagnosis of both untreated hyperthyroidism and methylphenidate given in excessive doses. The boy's presenting complaints are all features of ADHD, although many other specific symptoms and developmental characteristics are required before the diagnosis can be confirmed. It is recommended that a consultant child psychiatrist or community paediatrician make the diagnosis of ADHD. These individuals should also supervise management, which consists of behavioural modification strategies and drug treatment. Methylphenidate hydrochloride, an amphetamine derivative, is the first-line drug of choice for many cases of ADHD. It should be started at a low dosage and gradually increased until symptoms improve. If given in high doses nervousness, insomnia, headache, dizziness, tachycardia, hypertension, reduced appetite with weight loss and tremor can all occur. Other adverse effects include drowsiness, dyskinesia, poor growth, abdominal pain and nausea.

ANSWER 7.4

1. Serum alpha-fetoprotein
   Carcinoembryonic antigen
   IgG_2 levels
   DNA fragility testing
   Sweat test
   Mitogen proliferation studies
2. Ataxia telangiectasia

Ataxia telangiectasia presents with progressive ataxia, choreoathetosis, myoclonic jerking and oculomotor problems from early childhood. The associated telangiectases on the bulbar conjunctivae and other sun-exposed areas do not commonly present until after 3 years of age. Most affected children experience recurrent sinopulmonary problems. Immunologically, they have low levels of IgA, IgE and IgG_2, as well as a lymphopenia and poor proliferation to mitogen stimulation. Elevated alpha-fetoprotein and chromosomal breakage studies assist in the diagnosis.

ANSWER 7.5

1. Congenital central hypoventilation (CCHV, Ondine's curse)
   Delayed maturation of the respiratory control system
2. Ventilatory support ± progesterone

The story is characteristic of congenital central hypoventilation. Delayed maturation of the respiratory control system would be a possible alternative but the severity of the symptoms make it less likely. Differentiation is by

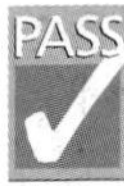

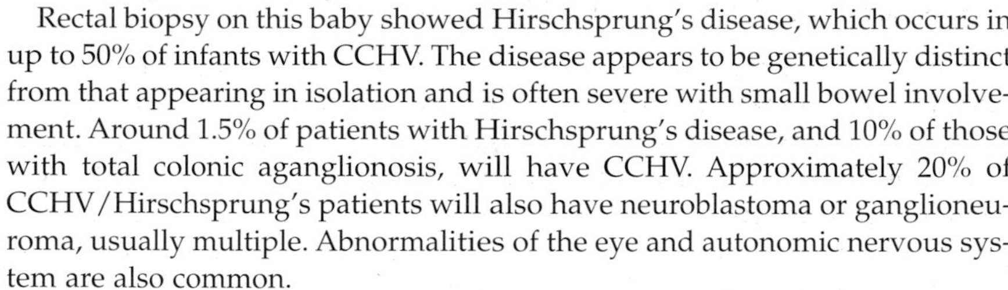

polygraphic sleep study, which shows a marked accentuation of the hypoventilation during quiet sleep. The natural history is usually for some improvement although all children continue to need ventilatory support during sleep. There may be a place for agents such as progesterone, which may increase chemoreceptor sensitivity to carbon dioxide.

Rectal biopsy on this baby showed Hirschsprung's disease, which occurs in up to 50% of infants with CCHV. The disease appears to be genetically distinct from that appearing in isolation and is often severe with small bowel involvement. Around 1.5% of patients with Hirschsprung's disease, and 10% of those with total colonic aganglionosis, will have CCHV. Approximately 20% of CCHV/Hirschsprung's patients will also have neuroblastoma or ganglioneuroma, usually multiple. Abnormalities of the eye and autonomic nervous system are also common.

Paper 8 *Questions*

8

QUESTION 8.1

An 18-month-old boy is referred by his GP because he has had diarrhoea and fever for 48 hours. The family returned from a rural part of The Gambia a week ago, where they had been visiting some friends who were missionaries. Whilst in The Gambia the family were taking malaria prophylaxis. The child is passing four watery, non-bloody stools per day and vomiting. On examination he is febrile (40.8°C), 5% dehydrated and lethargic. There is no lymphadenopathy or pallor. The chest is clear and there is no evidence of enlargement of abdominal organs. There is no meningism or irritability.

1. List three immediate investigations that you would perform.
2. What other investigations would you perform? List three.

QUESTION 8.2

A 6-year-old girl has been diagnosed with bilateral (Stage V) Wilms' tumour. No pulmonary metastases have been identified, and there is no intracaval extension of tumour. Her blood pressure was normal at presentation, and her admission neurological assessment was also unremarkable. She was treated with preoperative chemotherapy consisting of vincristine 1.5 mg/m^2 and actinomycin D 45 μg/kg on day 1 and vincristine 1.5 mg/m^2 alone on day 8. She developed mild jaw and lower extremity pain between her first two vincristine doses; these were relieved by analgesics. Three days after the second vincristine dose, she was admitted with constipation and worsening peripheral neuropathy. A further 3 days later she complained of not being able to see.

On examination, pupillary reflexes and fundoscopic examination were normal. During the examination she began to have seizure activity characterized by unresponsiveness, lip smacking, hypoventilation, conjugate eye deviation to the left, and right hand twitching. Her blood pressure was 154/91 mmHg. Cardiovascular and respiratory examination was normal. The seizure was controlled after administration of diazepam and phenytoin. The patient recovered fully.

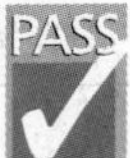

Serum urea and electrolytes	normal
Haemoglobin	9.2 g/dl
White cell count	$3.4 \times 10^9/l$
Platelets	$675 \times 10^9/l$
Prothrombin time	normal
Activated partial thromboplastin time	normal
CSF microscopy	1 white cell/mm^3, 31 red cells/mm^3
CSF protein	normal
CSF glucose	normal
CSF culture	negative
Blood culture	negative
CT head scan	normal
EEG	persistent interhemispheric asymmetry suggesting left cerebral dysfunction, possibly a postictal effect

1. What is the cause of this girl's neurological symptoms?
2. Suggest two investigations that may help confirm the cause of the blindness.
3. Suggest three other causes of blindness in this girl that need exclusion.

QUESTION 8.3

A 14-year-old boy was taken by his parents to the local Accident and Emergency department. He admitted to hearing a voice for the last 4 months. The voice was perceived to be inside his head. The patient commented that it had commanded him to undertake a series of acts, but initially would not disclose what these were. Later he admitted that the voice had ordered him to 'slash his thighs'. It had also repeatedly told him that he was 'no good' and 'really useless'.

His mother noted that her son had been more agitated and thought that he had lost weight. Many years ago his maternal grandfather was diagnosed as having schizophrenia. His brother has temporal lobe epilepsy, controlled with carbamazepine. On examination he had healing superficial lacerations to the lateral aspect of both thighs and mild flexural eczema. There were no neurological abnormalities. His blood pressure was 125/75 mmHg.

Haemoglobin	12.4 g/dl
White blood count	$6.1 \times 10^9/l$
Platelets	$147 \times 10^9/l$
Serum sodium	137 mmol/l
Serum potassium	4.5 mmol/l
Serum bicarbonate	22 mmol/l
Serum urea	4.7 mmol/l
Urine toxicology screen	negative
Thyroid function	normal
CT head scan	normal

1. What is the most likely diagnosis?

QUESTION 8.4

A 9-year-old boy presents with a 6-month history of recurrent abdominal pain. This has been episodic but has been more severe lately, waking him at night. His mother feels that he is now picking at his food but is uncertain of any significant weight loss. He looks pale during an episode and occasionally vomits. He often points to his upper abdomen as the site of the pain. He had an egg allergy as an infant but grew out of this by his fourth birthday. He had a perforated appendix removed last year. There is no history of travel sickness. He is on no medication at present. There is a family history of migraine. On examination, his weight and height are on the 75th centile. His blood pressure is 90/64 mmHg. Abdominal examination is unremarkable, with an appendix scar noted.

Haemoglobin	11.2 g/dl
White cell count	7.5×10^9/l
Platelets	301×10^9/l
ESR	4 mm/h
Liver function tests	normal
Urine microscopy	normal

1. What further two investigations would you do?
2. What is the diagnosis?
3. What is the management?

QUESTION 8.5

A 2-year-old girl was admitted to hospital with a 2-day history of fever and being generally unwell. In the last 12 hours she had complained that her head hurt. She had been born at term and had been previously well apart from having eczema, occasional wheezing and what her parents described as a 'constant cold'. On examination she was toxic and had meningism. Blood culture and CSF grew *Streptococcus pneumoniae*. She made an uneventful recovery after treatment with intravenous penicillin. A month later she was admitted with a similar story. Blood and CSF again grew *Streptococcus pneumoniae*. Examination of her ears was normal and a radiograph of her sinuses was clear. She was treated with penicillin, this time for 2 weeks.

Serum IgG	6.7 g/l (normal 3–11 g/l)
Serum IgM	1.1 g/l (normal 0.3–1.4 g/l)
Serum IgA	0.5 g/l (normal 0.5–2 g/l)
Complement C3	1.6 g/l (normal 0.68–1.8 g/l)
Complement C4	0.6 g/l (normal 0.18–0.6 g/l)

Three months later she presented again with pneumococcal meningitis.

1. What are the most likely reasons for the recurrent infection?
2. How would you investigate her further?

Paper 8 *Answers*

8

ANSWER 8.1

1. Blood glucose
   Serum urea and electrolytes
   Thin film for malaria parasites
2. Full blood count
   Blood culture
   Stool culture

Malaria is the most pressing disease to exclude and a series of three blood films should be made. Other clues may be anaemia and elevated serum bilirubin. This child had malaria, for which the main presenting symptom was fever together with the history of travel to an endemic area. Diarrhoea is common with malaria. Malaria can be contracted even when correctly taking malaria prophylaxis. As in this case, prophylaxis is usually not taken correctly. Treatment should continue for at least 4 weeks after return but was stopped in this case on the family's return to the UK. Any febrile illness within 3 months of return from a malaria-endemic area should prompt investigations for malaria. Glucose should be checked in a lethargic child. Possible diagnoses other than malaria include gastroenteritis. With a high fever consideration of *Shigella* or *Salmonella* septicaemia should be made.

ANSWER 8.2

1. Vincristine-associated transient blindness and neurotoxicity
2. Electro-retinogram
   Cerebral MRI scan
3. Trauma
   Hypertension
   Direct extension or metastatic spread of malignancy to the occipital region
   Hypoxia induced by seizures

Cortical blindness refers to loss of sight due to injury to the occipital lobes, with intact pupillary reflexes and normal retinal examination, as in the

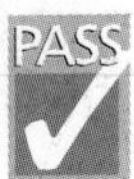

patient presented here. Cortical blindness may result from trauma, cerebrovascular compromise due to cardiac disease, instrumentation such as angiography, as a post-perfusion phenomenon, from hypertension, from direct extension or metastatic spread of malignancy to the occipital region, or from hypoxia induced by seizures. Drug-induced cortical blindness is a rarely reported clinical entity: cisplatin and vincristine are the two chemotherapeutics previously cited as potential causative agents.

In this case, other aetiologies for transient blindness and seizures are incompatible with the clinical course. The concomitant findings of additional significant vincristine neurotoxicity and, most importantly, a temporal relationship to rechallenge with vincristine, strongly suggest that vincristine administration was the most likely aetiology of the neurological symptoms. Magnetic resonance imaging (MRI) may be a particularly useful diagnostic tool in evaluating patients with transient cortical blindness; cranial computed tomography may not reveal the typical occipital lobe changes associated with this syndrome, while MRI can demonstrate the pathology clearly. MRI may demonstrate focal areas of hyperintense signal in the occipital lobes bilaterally involving both the cortical and subcortical regions.

ANSWER 8.3

1. Severe depression

This young man has many of the features of severe depression. He has auditory hallucinations of a derogatory nature that instructed him to commit self-harm. These commanding hallucinations are associated with severe depression and contrast with the third-person running commentary that is seen in schizophrenia or the musical hallucinations of temporal lobe epilepsy. He also has agitation and associated weight loss. Often in cases of this severity there is a family history of depression. This patient's grandfather was originally labelled as schizophrenic although it is likely that he would currently be considered to have schizo-affective disorder.

Other features of serious depression include: psychomotor retardation and apathy, early morning wakening, insomnia or hypersomnia, feelings of worthlessness or helplessness, an inability to concentrate, crying spells or the inability to cry and diminished interest or pleasure in most activities. Recurrent or persistent psychosomatic complaints such as abdominal or chest pain, dizziness or headache may also be present. Many drugs may cause depressive symptoms, including ecstasy, cocaine, phenylcyclidine and withdrawal from amphetamines. It is important that drug misuse is excluded as a cause for this patient's history.

ANSWER 8.4

1. Endoscopy and antral biopsy
   CLO (urease) test/microbiological culture of antral specimen
2. Peptic ulcer disease (probably associated with *Helicobacter pylori* gastritis)

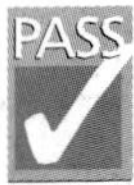

3. Prolonged treatment with H_2 antagonist/proton pump inhibitor
   Eradication therapy with triple treatment
   Follow-up repeat C^{13} urea breath test

Recurrent abdominal pain can have both organic and non-organic origins in childhood. More convincing symptoms of organic origin are pain away from the periumbilical region, nocturnal wakening and bilious vomiting. Abdominal migraine is often a diagnosis of exclusion, though a strong history of travel sickness and a family history of migraine will support the diagnosis. A CLO test is dependent on the urease-splitting properties of *Helicobacter pylori* that change the colour of the small specimen well.

ANSWER 8.5

1. Communication with CSF space
2. Detection of CSF leak, neuroimaging

The volume and sugar content of her nasal discharge was estimated by leaving cotton wool pledgets up her nose overnight. These were stained with a small quantity of clear fluid containing 4 mmol/l glucose. MRI revealed a defect in the cribriform plate allowing a direct communication to the CSF space. Surgical closure of the defect prevented further episodes.

Paper 9 *Questions*

9

QUESTION 9.1

A 1-year-old boy is a recent refugee immigrant from West Africa. He presents with a 4-week history of watery diarrhoea and weight loss. The child has been in the UK for 2 weeks and before the onset of diarrhoea was said to be well. On examination the child was underweight (z-score –3.0) and stunted (height z-score –2.5), less than 5% dehydrated but afebrile. The rest of the examination was unremarkable.

Stool culture and microscopy	negative (× 3)
Haemoglobin	9.4 g/dl
White cell count	$6.5 \times 10^9/l$
Platelets	$322 \times 10^9/l$
MCV	90 fl
Serum urea and electrolytes	normal
IgG	13 g/l (age-appropriate upper limit of normal 8 g/l)

1. What investigations would you perform? (List 5)
2. What is the significance of the low haemoglobin and high MCV?

QUESTION 9.2

A 14-month-old boy presents with a 5-month history of cradle cap and a rash on his back that have been unresponsive to general skin care, 1% hydrocortisone cream and topical antifungals (see Fig. 9.1). The rash has looked haemorrhagic at times, and eczematous at others. He has a family history of psoriasis (mother and a maternal uncle) and eczema (older sister had moderately severe eczema as a baby). In addition, the boy has a persistent 'ear infection' affecting his right ear, but this has not responded to topical or systemic antibiotics. He is otherwise well and no other abnormalities are evident on examination. There is a sero-sanguinous discharge from his ear but the tympanic membrane itself is obscured. The left ear is normal.

1. What is the diagnosis?
2. Which other organs can be affected?

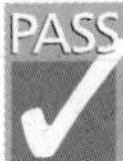

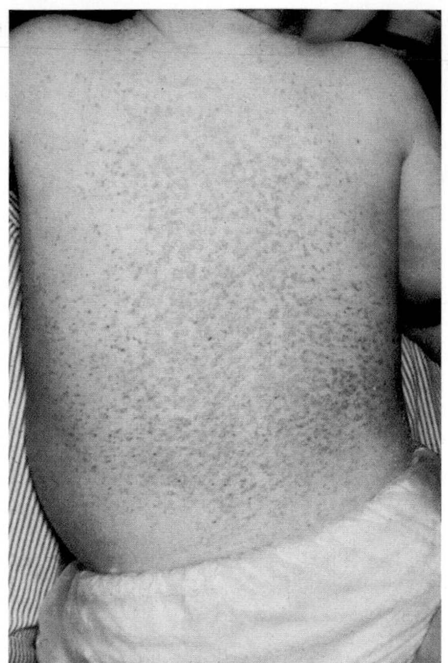

Fig. 9.1

QUESTION 9.3

A 9-week-old baby boy was referred because his mother was concerned that he was not smiling. He was born by spontaneous vertex delivery at term, weighing 2800 g. He required active resuscitation at birth but was subsequently transferred to the postnatal ward. He had bottle fed well and gained weight appropriately but had been constipated. His mother had type 1 diabetes and there was a family history of epilepsy. On examination he did not appear to visually fix or follow and either looked around randomly or occasionally at the brightest light in the room. Nystagmus was absent. His development was otherwise normal. A full neurological assessment including fundoscopy was normal.

Electroretinogram	within normal limits
Visual evoked potentials	within normal limits

1. What is the most likely diagnosis?
2. What is the prognosis for this condition?

QUESTION 9.4

A 15-year-old boy has been complaining of dysuria and urinary frequency for the last 3 weeks. He had seen his GP after the first week of the problem, who had taken a MSU and commenced him on trimethoprim. The MSU has subsequently been reported as no growth. As an infant, he had had balanitis xerotica obliterans and had a circumcision preformed. He is general fit and well. He is a keen rower and is in the county Under-18 team. His 48-year-old father has hypertension that is controlled by medication. His younger brother is under investigation for recurrent headaches. On examination, he is afebrile. His weight and height are both above the 97th centile. His blood pressure is 122/74 mmHg. Abdominal examination is normal. Fundoscopy is normal.

Serum sodium	141 mmol/l
Serum potassium	4.0 mmol/l
Serum urea	3.4 mmol/l
Serum creatinine	72 μmol/l
Urinary protein/creatinine ratio	normal
Urinary microscopy	non-glomerular red cells and white cells seen, no organisms

1. What three other investigation would you do?
2. What is the diagnosis?
3. List three further management steps.

QUESTION 9.5

A male infant weighing 3575 g was born to a 28-year-old primigravida. Delivery was by forceps rotation for persistent occipito-posterior position. Apgar scores were 2 at 1 minute and 5 at 5 minutes. He was intubated at 1 minute for 5 minutes, after which he breathed normally on his own and remained pink in air. The paediatrician was asked to review him on the postnatal ward at 6 hours of age because he was noted to have noisy breathing. On examination he was slightly cyanosed with a heart rate of 170/min and a respiratory rate of 60/min. There was a grade 2 systolic murmur at the apex and his liver was palpable 5 cm below the right costal margin. The baby was transferred to the regional cardiac unit for further investigation. At the cardiac unit he was noted in addition to have full pulses and a hyperdynamic precordium.

Chest radiograph	cardiomegaly with increased pulmonary vasculature
Echocardiogram	normal structure; large right atrium with high volume return from the superior vena cava; left ventricular overload
ECG	Fig. 9.2

1. What do the above findings suggest?
2. What are the possible aetiologies?
3. Suggest two other investigations that might assist diagnosis.

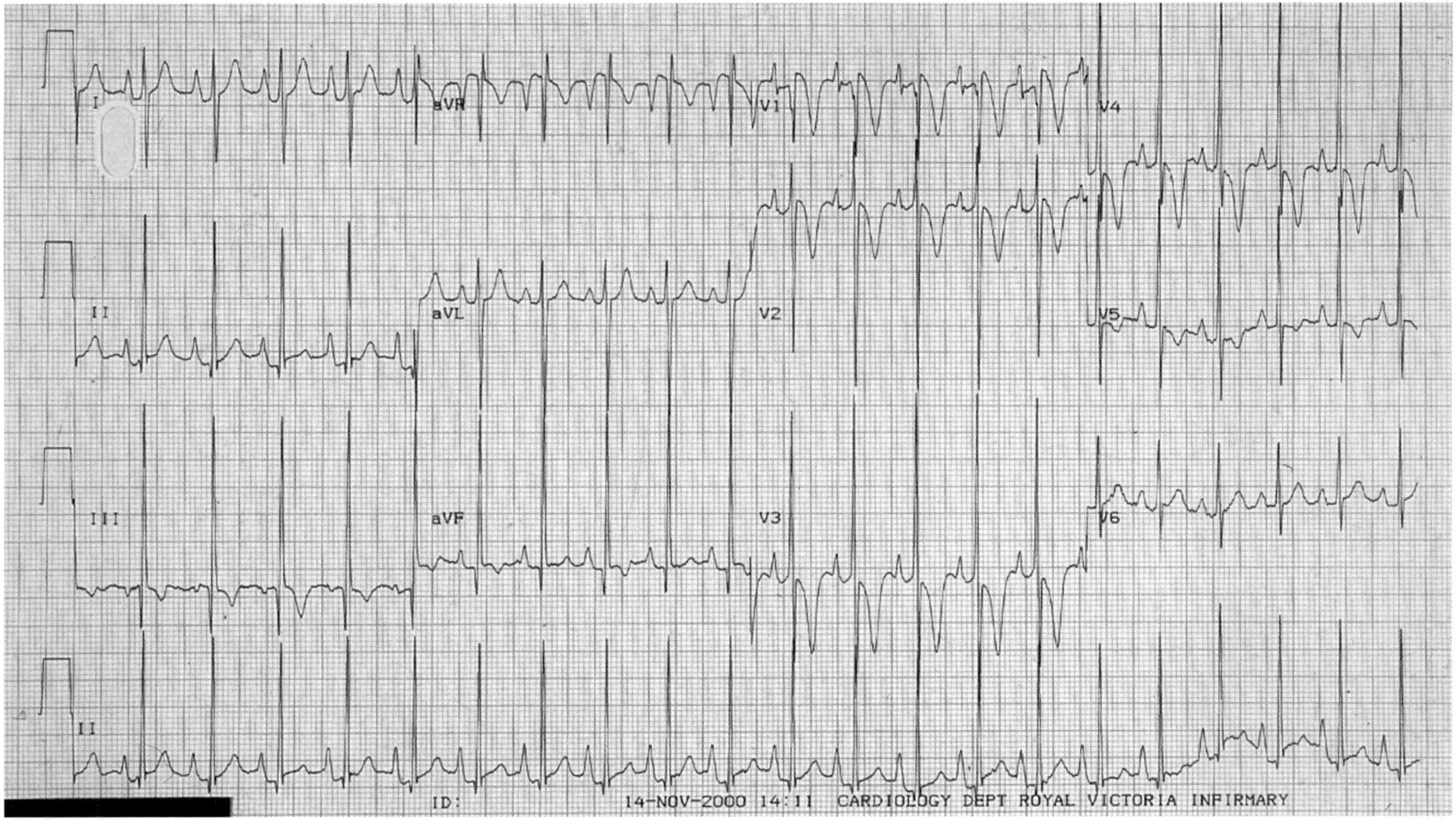

I aVR V1 V4
II aVL V2 V5
III aVF V3 V6
II
ID: 14-NOV-2000 14:11 CARDIOLOGY DEPT ROYAL VICTORIA INFIRMARY

Fig. 9.2

Paper 9 *Answers*

9

ANSWER 9.1

1. Stool microscopy using modified Ziehl–Nielson stain
   Stool electron microscopy
   Coeliac antibody screen
   Small bowel biopsy
   HIV screen
2. Nutritional deprivation or malabsorption

This child had *Cryptosporidium parvum* infection. There is no way of knowing this from the history, but some clues are given. Firstly in the tropics *C. parvum* is not a rare disease, causing acute or chronic diarrhoea. The other intestinal parasite to consider is *Giardia lamblia*, but this will usually be detected by finding either cysts or trophozoites in the stool by simple microscopy. *Cryptosporidium* requires a special stain to identify its presence. The other relevant investigations are a small bowel biopsy (this produces a higher diagnostic yield for intestinal parasites than faecal microscopy, and some Ethiopian tribes are known to suffer from coeliac disease), and stool electron microscopy for microsporidium.

A moderately elevated MCV and anaemia of this order is compatible with nutritional deprivation or a degree of malabsorption. Steatorrhoea does not occur if there is a low-fat diet, as is the case for most children from poor areas of Africa. Raised immunoglobulins (all subclasses) are seen in children from the tropics and our reference ranges do not apply.

ANSWER 9.2

1. Class I histiocytosis (Langerhans histiocytosis, histiocytosis X)
2. Bone
   Bone marrow
   Lymph nodes
   Liver
   Lungs
   Pituitary
   Spleen

Histiocytosis is a heterogeneous group of disorders. Class I histiocytosis (Langerhans cell histiocytosis or histiocytosis X) is the largest group and encompasses the entities formerly known as eosinophilic granuloma, Hand–Schüeller–Christian triad and Letterer–Siwe disease. These conditions present in a variety of ways from non-specific aches and pains to bone lesions, widespread lymphadenopathy, hepatosplenomegaly and skin rash. Chronic otitis media, diabetes insipidus and weight loss are seen with some types. Treatment depends on the stage of disease and evidence of progression. Local lesions may be treated with local excision and irradiation and graded use of chemotherapy in stage III disease. Class I histiocytosis responds to steroids in 90% of cases but there is a high relapse rate.

ANSWER 9.3

1. Delayed visual maturation
2. Excellent for sight. A few children develop minor neurological problems in later life

Delayed visual maturation is characterised by visual unresponsiveness in early infancy that improves spontaneously to normal levels by 6–12 months of age. Ocular examination, visual evoked potentials and the electroretinogram are usually normal. It is due primarily to a subcortical defect, which secondarily delays the emergence of cortically mediated visual responses.

It can present as an idiopathic isolated abnormality (as illustrated by this case) or be associated with perinatal problems; severe generalised neurodevelopmental delay, maternal cocaine abuse or ocular abnormalities. This last is commonly associated with nystagmus. Isolated delayed visual maturation usually has an extremely good neurological prognosis. However, it can be associated with the later development of mild autism, clumsiness and hypotonia.

ANSWER 9.4

1. Direct swabbing of anterior urethra
   Urinary PCR for chlamydia
   Direct fluorescent test of urethral discharge
2. Non-specific urethritis
3. Antibiotic therapy (dependent on isolation and sensitivity of particular organism)
   Contact tracing
   Opportune sexual education particularly about pregnancy sexually transmitted diseases, HIV and Hepatitis B, and the usage of condoms.

This boy presents with symptoms of urethritis though did not disclose a history of urethral discharge. Sexual practice is now more common in the teenage population with an increase in pregnancy and sexual transmitted diseases. Teenagers whose peer group is older are more likely to develop adult practices earlier.

ANSWER 9.5

1. High-output cardiac failure
2. Low-resistance shunt (for example arteriovenous malformation or abnormal venoarterial connections)
3. Cranial ultrasound
   Angiography

The baby had typical signs of high-output cardiac failure. There are no obvious cardiac reasons for the condition and it is possible that there is a low-resistance arteriovenous shunt elsewhere. The large volume of blood returning to the right atrium from the superior vena cava suggests that the shunt is in the head and neck. External inspection revealed no abnormalities but auscultation of the head revealed a loud continuous bruit, maximal posteriorly. Ultrasound of the brain showed an aneurysm of the vein of Galen with high flow. The diagnosis was confirmed with MRI and angiography. Treatment of this type of arteriovenous malformation may be possible using embolisation but the outlook for intact neurological function remains poor because of the regional cortical 'steal' by the large shunt in utero.

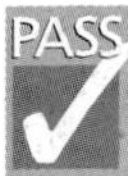

Paper 10 *Questions*

10

QUESTION 10.1

A 3-month-old girl is brought to the Accident and Emergency department for the third time in 3 weeks with feeding difficulties. She is the first child of a single unsupported 17-year-old mother. The mother says that the baby appears hungry but as soon as she has taken a small amount of feed she develops severe colic and refuses to feed further. Because she has been feeding so poorly over the last month she has lost weight. The first time she presented to hospital she was admitted overnight but no cause was found for her symptoms.

On examination she is pink in air but appears sweaty. Her weight is on the 10th centile, having previously been on the 25th centile from birth. There is a holosystolic murmur heard best at the apex. Her femoral pulses are palpable.

CXR	mild cardiomegaly, pulmonary venous engorgement
ECG	Fig. 10.1

1. What does the ECG show?
2. What is the diagnosis?

QUESTION 10.2

An 8-year-old with type 1 diabetes mellitus has been attending outpatients since her initial diagnosis at the age of 3 years. Generally her diabetic control has been acceptable. During the past 7 months her control has been somewhat erratic. At the last clinic 3 months ago her HbA1c was 7.9%. She does not report any unusual symptoms and says that she has been following all the dietary advice. Her diary shows a mixture of hypoglycaemic and hyperglycaemic blood sugar estimations. Her growth chart is shown (Fig. 10.2):

HbA1c	8.2%
Haemoglobin	9.4 g/dl
White cell count	normal
Platelets	normal
T_4	97 nmol/l (normal 60–160 nmol/l)
Bone age estimation	6.4 years (chronological age 8.5 years)

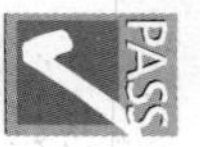

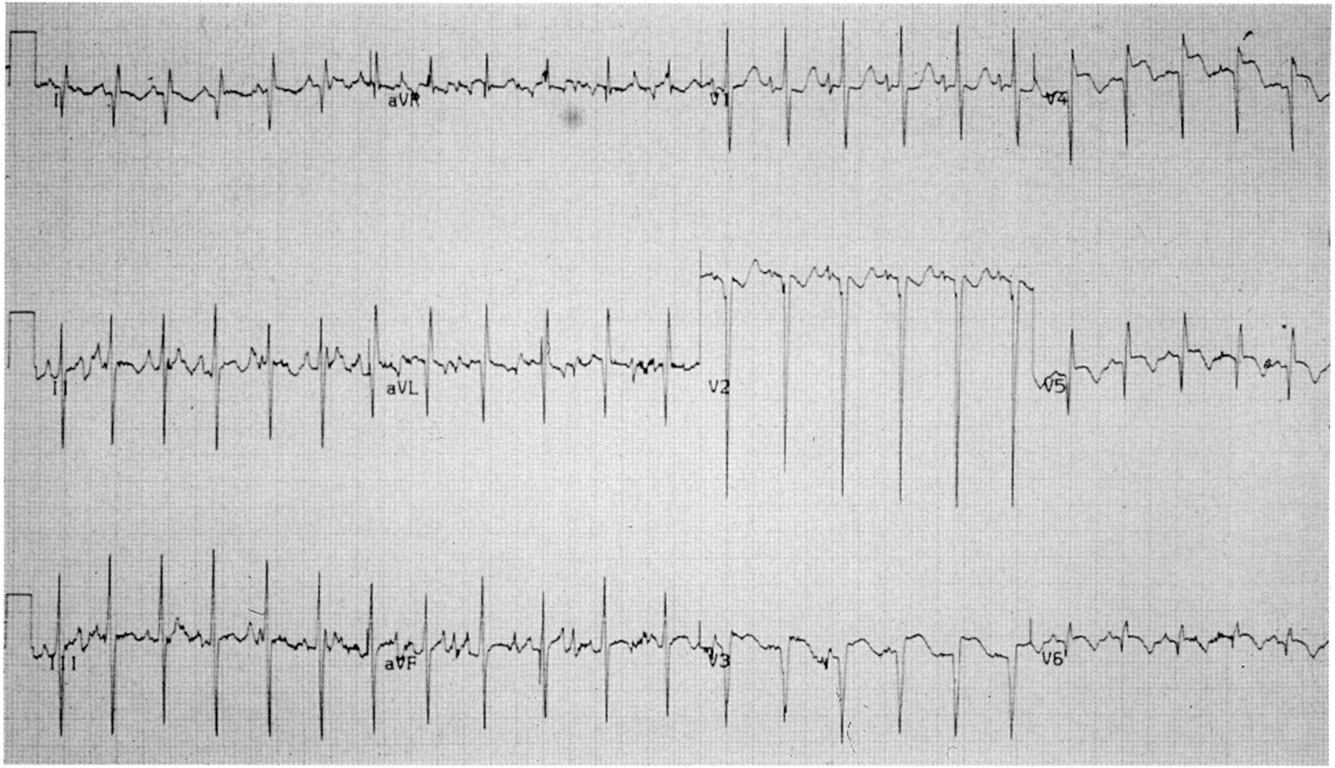

Fig. 10.1

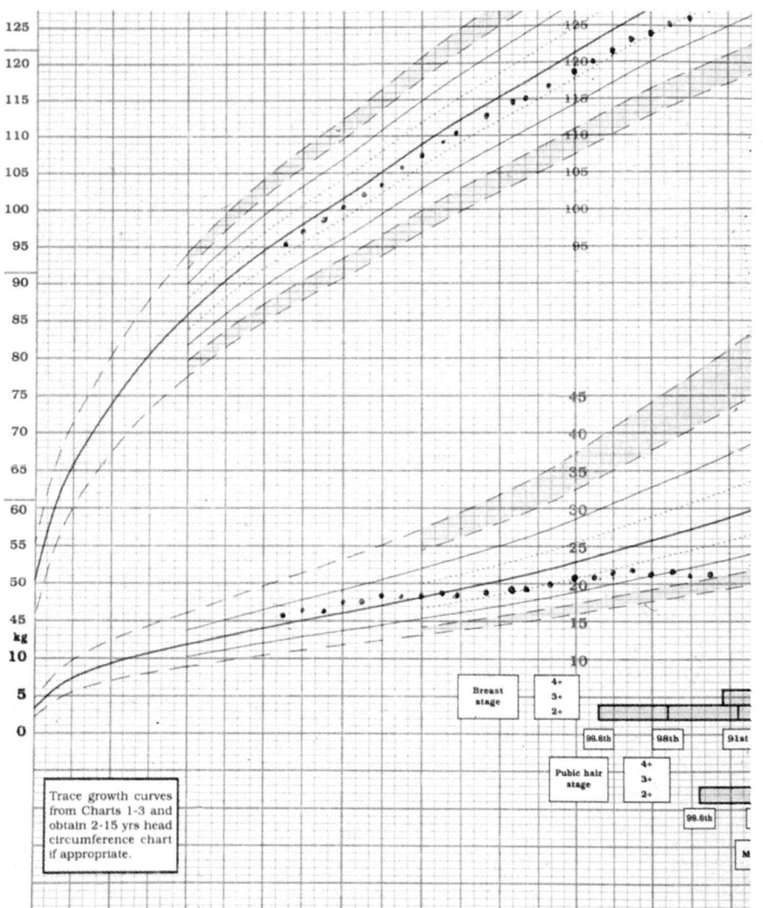

Fig. 10.2

1. What is the diagnosis, and the cause for this girl's poor diabetic control and growth?
2. What other blood test would you consider performing?
3. What other test will confirm the diagnosis?
4. What changes to her management are needed?

QUESTION 10.3

A 7-year-old girl was reviewed after she developed gross macroscopic haematuria after a sore throat and upper respiratory tract infection. She had no urinary symptoms but felt she had passed less urine than usual. She complained of mild diffuse lower abdominal pain. Her past medical history was unremarkable other than that she had suffered with intermittent headaches for the last 2 years. There was a family history of haemochromatosis.

On examination she appeared to be well and her blood pressure was 95/65 mmHg. No oedema was present. A degree of suprapubic tenderness was noted on abdominal examination. Review of her ear, nose and throat revealed that she was coryzal with red tympanic membranes bilaterally and inflamed fauces.

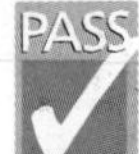

Serum sodium	136 mmol/l
Serum potassium	4.8 mmol/l
Serum bicarbonate	24 mmol/l
Serum urea	6.2 mmol/l
Serum creatinine	47 μmol/l
Prothrombin time	14 s (control 11–15 s)
Activated partial thromboplastin time	23 s (control 24–35 s)
Fibrinogen	3.7 g/l (normal 1.5–4.0 g/l)
Urine dipstick	+++ blood, no protein
Urine culture	no growth

Her macroscopic haematuria settled but she continued to have +++ blood on urine dipstick testing. She was re-referred by her GP 3 months later with a further diagnosed episode of glomerulonephritis. She had again developed macroscopic haematuria after a coryzal illness.

1. What is the most likely diagnosis?
2. List six further investigations that would help confirm the diagnosis.
3. What is her renal prognosis?

QUESTION 10.4

A 7-year-old girl presents to the Accident and Emergency department complaining of difficulties in blinking and persistent drooling from the left side of her mouth. She had been seen in the past by her GP with recurrent upper respiratory tract infections and fevers but has had no recent attendances. She appears to be an accident–prone girl, having recently broken her right forearm for the second time this year. Her younger sister has chickenpox but appears quite well. There is no other family history of note.

On examination, her weight is on the 9th centile and her height is on the 3rd centile. When she tries to smile or frown, she has no facial creases on the left side of her face. Examination of her ears, nose and throat is unremarkable. Fundoscopy shows two small haemorrhages in the temporal region of the right eye. Full neurological examination is otherwise normal. Her chest is clinically clear, with normal heart sounds on auscultation. Palpation of her abdomen is unremarkable.

Haemoglobin	9.2 g/dl
White cell count	6.4×10^9/l
Platelets	259×10^9/l
Serum sodium	136 mmol/l
Serum potassium	5.5 mmol/l
Serum urea	12.3 mmol/l
Serum creatinine	332 μmol/l
Alkaline phosphatase	663 IU/l
Serum calcium	1.99 mmol/l
Serum phosphate	1.66 mmol/l

1. List one immediate investigation.
2. List six further investigations.
3. What is the underlying diagnosis?

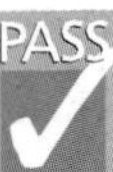

QUESTION 10.5

A 1-year-old boy presented with a 5-day history of swelling of his fingers. The swelling had appeared overnight and during the subsequent 5 days had not changed. During this time the affected fingers had taken on a bluish discoloration. He had been otherwise well both before and during this time, apart from a cough which had persisted since a 'flu-like illness 2 months earlier. There had been no fever, rash, systemic upset or obvious pain. He was the middle of triplets born at 32 weeks and had been ventilated for 3 days for mild surfactant deficiency lung disease. His siblings had been well. There was no significant family history. His mother thought that the hands of all three triplets felt a little cold in the mornings.

On examination he was very well and smiled and played happily with the examiner. A photograph of his hands is shown below (Fig. 10.3). The fingers were a normal temperature and there was no obvious pain. Clinical examination was otherwise unremarkable apart from mild eczema.

1. What is the most likely diagnosis?
2. How would you confirm this?

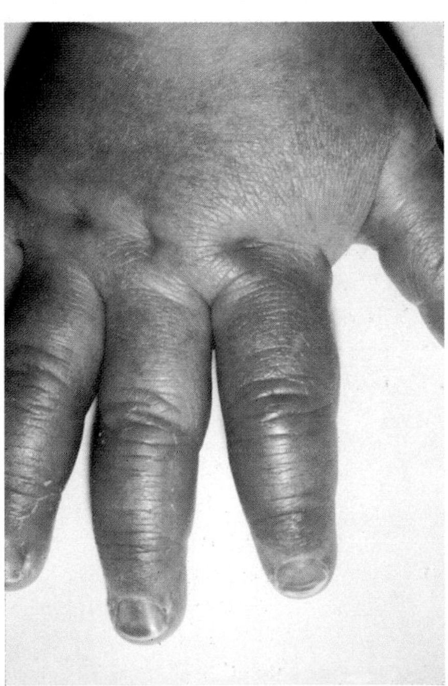

Fig. 10.3

Paper 10 *Answers*

10

ANSWER 10.1

1. Anterolateral myocardial infarct
2. Anomalous origin of coronary artery

Anomalous origin of the coronary arteries is rare. Anomalies include the location, number and patency of the coronary ostia in addition to the course of the primary portions of the coronary arteries. The most important clinical variant is when the left coronary artery arises from the pulmonary trunk. Distal anomalies include total or partial intramural courses of the coronary arteries or fistulae (arteriovenous, or between the artery and either myocardial sinuses or cardiac chambers). The resulting symptoms of angina may present in infancy as pain (often associated with pallor or sweating) on feeding. Older children who have adequate collateral circulation may have normal cardiac findings apart from mitral regurgitation. The murmur in this case was due to mitral regurgitation as a result of papillary muscle ischaemia. Treatment is reimplantation of the coronary artery, which if successful nearly always produces recovery of ventricular function.

ANSWER 10.2

1. Coeliac disease
2. Screening for coeliac disease
3. Jejunal biopsy
4. She will need a combined gluten-free and diabetic diet

The prevalence of coeliac disease in type 1 diabetes mellitus is higher than in the general population, with estimates ranging from 2 to 10%. IgG antigliadin, IgA antigliadin and IgA antiendomysial antibodies were all strongly positive in this girl. Many patients with coeliac disease are asymptomatic. Typical gastrointestinal complaints of coeliac disease (such as diarrhoea, abdominal distension) are rare in type I diabetes, while atypical isolated signs or symptoms are more common; in particular anaemia, short stature, delayed puberty, epilepsy, dyspeptic symptoms, herpetiform dermatitis and recurrent

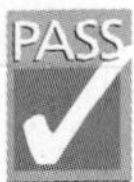

aphthous stomatitis. Consideration should be given to performing an annual coeliac disease screen on all patients with type 1 diabetes.

ANSWER 10.3

1. IgA nephropathy (Berger's disease)
   Reject: Post-streptococcal glomerulonephritis
2. Ultrasound scan of renal tract
   Urine microscopy
   C3 and C4
   Urinary protein/creatinine ratio
   Plasma IgA
   Full blood count
3. Very good

This patient has IgA nephropathy and not post-streptococcal glomerulonephritis (PSGN). She developed recurrent macroscopic haematuria without proteinuria after coryzal illnesses, a characteristic feature of Berger's disease. In cases of PSGN there is usually a history of a sore throat 7–10 days before the onset of glomerulonephritis, evidence of circulatory overload with mild peripheral oedema and some proteinuria with macroscopic haematuria (which is seldom gross). Recurrences of PSGN are never seen.

IgA nephropathy is a disease whose onset is usually between 5 and 10 years of age. It affects boys twice as commonly as girls and is characterised by recurrent episodes of macroscopic haematuria usually precipitated by upper respiratory tract infections. Most children are normotensive and have normal urine or microscopic haematuria between bouts of macroscopic bleeding. Proteinuria is usually absent. Complement studies are normal and in some individuals the serum IgA is elevated. Overall, the prognosis in this condition is good. However, approximately 20% of all children affected will have a significant deterioration in renal function, usually in adult life. Poor prognostic indicators include being older than 10 years of age at presentation, the presence of heavy proteinuria, a reduced glomerular filtration rate, hypertension and the absence of macroscopic haematuria. This patient had none of these.

Additional, but less appropriate, investigations include further plasma biochemistry, antinuclear antibodies (ANA), antineutrophil cytoplasmic antibodies (ANCA), antistreptolysin O titre (ASOT) and family screening for haematuria.

ANSWER 10.4

1. Blood pressure with an appropriate sized cuff.
2. Renal tract ultrasound
   DMSA scan
   Radiograph of wrist
   Echocardiogram
   Micturating cystourethrogram
   Parathyroid hormone level

3. Chronic renal failure with secondary hypertension and osteodystrophy

An isolated facial palsy may be the presenting symptom of hypertension. This girl's chronic renal failure is secondary to reflux nephropathy and occult urinary tract infection in infancy. The systemic hypertension and bone disease are secondary to this.

ANSWER 10.5

1. Raynaud's phenomenon associated with cold agglutinins following mycoplasma infection
2. Measure cold agglutinins

Symptoms associated with cold agglutinin formation after mycoplasma infection are uncommon but well documented. They usually affect the peripheries and last for several months. Severity ranges from mild to those with Raynaud's-type phenomena. It is not clear whether this was a feature in this case. Treatment is expectant unless tissue viability is at risk, when steroids may accelerate recovery.

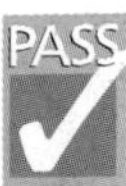

Paper 11 *Questions*

11

QUESTION 11.1

A female infant was born at 36 weeks' gestation, birthweight 1540 g, being the first child of healthy unrelated parents. Pregnancy had been uneventful until the week before delivery when the fetus had been felt to be small for gestational age. Investigations had revealed oligohydramnios and cardiomegaly and a poor fetal biophysical profile. This had prompted delivery by Caesarean section. At delivery the infant needed active resuscitation, including intubation and ventilation. She was pale and had mild elbow contractures but there were no other abnormal findings or dysmorphic features. Investigations were as follows:

Haemoglobin	2.7 g/dl
White blood count	$5.8 \times 10^9/l$
Platelets	$35 \times 10^9/l$
Infant's blood group	A positive
Coombs test	negative
Maternal Kleihauer	negative
Echocardiogram	normal connections, right ventricular hypertrophy

She was transfused, her ventilatory status improved and she was extubated. Over the following 4 weeks she showed poor growth despite adequate milk intake, became repeatedly anaemic requiring transfusion and remained thrombocytopenic. She also became persistently neutropenic and developed insulin-dependent diabetes. TORCH and parvovirus serology were negative. A blood film was performed (Fig. 11.1(i), (ii)):

1. What abnormalities are shown on the film?
2. Suggest a possible diagnosis.
3. What investigations would you perform?

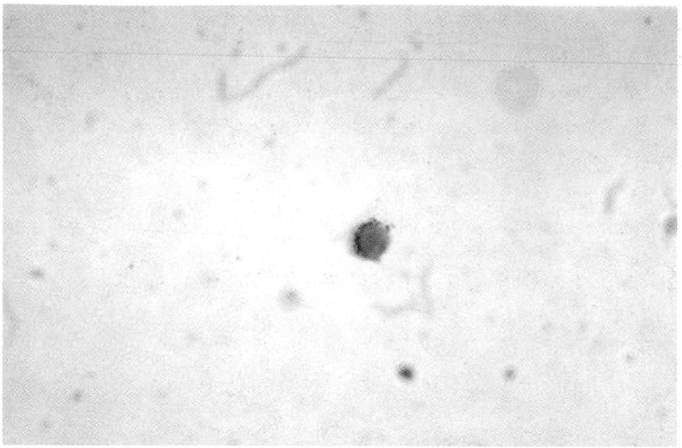

Fig. 11.1(i)

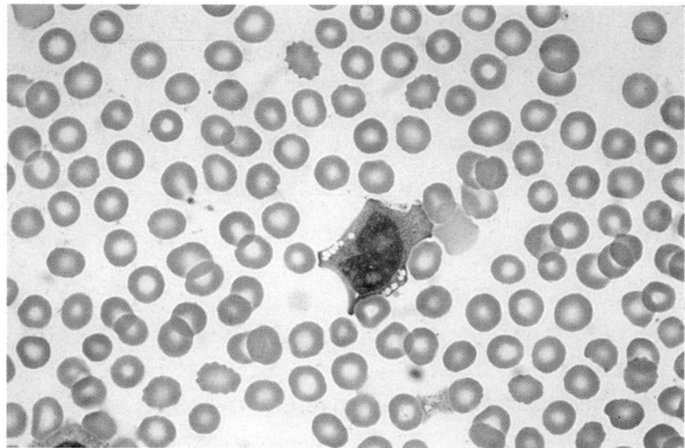

Fig. 11.1(ii)

QUESTION 11.2

A 6-year-old girl is referred by her GP with breast development. She has been previously well. She was born at term by normal delivery with subsequent normal development. Her weight and height have only been intermittently measured but she has always been one of the tallest in her class. She was previously admitted to hospital at the age of 8 months with suspected meningitis but prior treatment with antibiotics meant no organism was isolated. A hearing test was normal but she defaulted from further follow-up. She lives with her mother who recalls her own periods began at the age of 13 years.

Examination shows a healthy girl. Her height is on the 97th centile and weight on the 90th centile. There are no birth marks or neurocutaneous stigmata. Cardiac and respiratory systems are normal. She has breast development equivalent to Tanner stage B3+ and sparse pubic hairs (Tanner stage PH2+). She also has enlargement of the labia minora.

Bone age	10.2 years (chronological age 6.1 years)
Skull radiograph	normal
Pelvic ultrasound	enlargement of the uterus and multicystic appearance of both ovaries
Serum oestradiol	elevated
LH & FSH	elevated
Thyroid function tests	normal

1. What is the cause of this girl's precocious puberty?
2. How may this be confirmed?
3. What other investigation might be considered?
4. What is the treatment and why is this considered?

QUESTION 11.3

A 9-year-old girl was admitted with a 4-week history of increasing lethargy and vomiting. Her lethargy prevented her from staying at school after midday. She was sleeping for most of the afternoon as well as through the night. She vomited three or four times each day, usually before meals. There were no other precipitating factors. The vomitus was yellow. Her mother has depression and takes tricyclic anti-depressants.

Five months previously she had presented with steroid-resistant nephrotic syndrome. A renal biopsy at that time demonstrated focal segmental glomerulosclerosis. She was treated with a 12-week course of oral cyclophosphamide and prednisolone followed by steroids alone for the last 8 weeks. On examination she had very mild ankle oedema and was normotensive. She was orientated and alert with no focal neurological signs. Examination of her cranial nerves was normal other than the presence of convergent nystagmus. On fundoscopy her optic disc margins were blurred.

Haemoglobin	12.6 g/dl
White blood count	$8.3 \times 10^9/l$
Platelets	$347 \times 10^9/l$
ESR	35 mm/h
Serum sodium	133 mmol/l
Serum potassium	3.8 mmol/l
Serum urea	15.0 mmol/l
Serum creatinine	93 μmol/l
Serum albumin	16 g/l
EEG	normal

1. What are the two most likely diagnoses?
2. What investigation differentiates between these?

QUESTION 11.4

A 12-year-old boy is referred with recurrent right hypochondrial pain. This has been intermittent and dull in nature. He has otherwise been well. He has refused to take part in PE at school recently. As a toddler, he had a

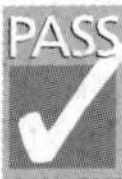

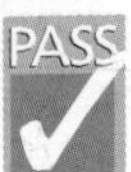

urinary tract infection and screening showed a small scar on the pole of the left kidney. His blood pressure has been monitored annually and it was previously noted as normal. His 7-year old sister is a well-controlled type 1 diabetic. On examination his weight is well above the 97th centile, with his height on the 75th centile. There is a pigmented area on the left side of his neck (Fig. 11.2) but he has no goitre. His blood pressure is 130/74 mmHg. On palpation of his abdomen, his liver edge is 2 cm palpable below the right costal margin. There is no splenomegaly. Testicular volume is 12 ml.

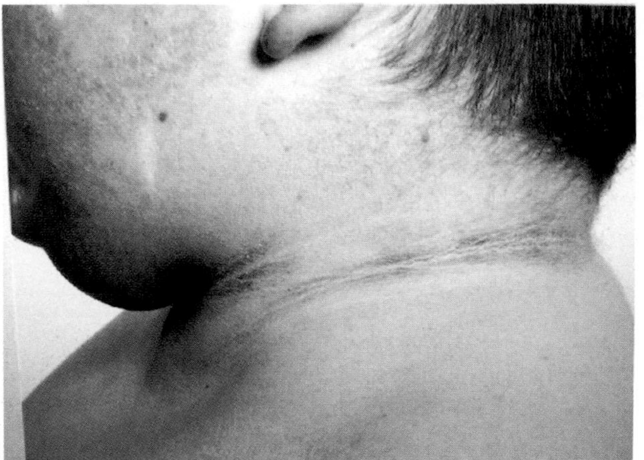

Fig. 11.2

Serum protein	61 g/l
Serum albumin	39 g/l
Aspartate transaminase	110 IU/l (normal 10–45 IU/l)
Alanine transaminase	196 IU/l (normal 0–25 IU/l)
Alkaline phosphatase	344 IU/l
Serum bilirubin	28 μmol/l
Coagulation screen	normal
Hepatitis serology	negative
Autoantibody screen	negative
Serum ceruloplasmin	normal
Fasting cholesterol	4.5 mmol/l (normal 3.2–4.4 mmol/l)
Fasting triglycerides	1.4 mmol/l (normal 0.35–1.60 mmol/l)
Random blood glucose	5.6 mmol/l
Abdominal ultrasound	increased echogenicity of the liver, left kidney smaller and slightly asymmetrical compared with right kidney

1. What is the diagnosis?
2. What is the management?

QUESTION 11.5

An 18-week-old baby girl is referred with a rash on her chin and the back of her head. This had started as very small erythematous lesions which had subsequently coalesced. The rash had failed to respond to a proprietary cream that contained an antifungal and hydrocortisone, and treatment with a topical antibiotic resulted in only minimal improvement. She had been born at 27 weeks' gestation, birthweight 1050 g, following an antepartum haemorrhage. She required mechanical ventilation for 6 days after birth and was extubated onto CPAP for a further week. She required parenteral nutrition until she was tolerating full enteral feeds (day 14). This comprised 50% expressed breast milk, 50% preterm formula until full breast feeding was established at 36 weeks' corrected gestation. Her neonatal course was otherwise uneventful apart from an episode of candidal nappy rash and chronic lung disease requiring home oxygen. Her 3-year-old sister had recently been treated for impetigo. Her parents were both healthy although there was a strong family history of atopy. Examination revealed an erythematous rash on her chin (Fig. 11.3) and a mild nappy rash. Her weight was 3760 g.

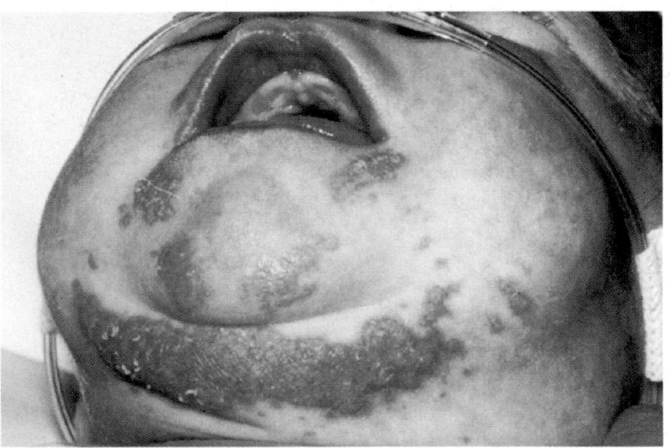

Fig. 11.3

1. Suggest a diagnosis.
2. What investigation would you perform?
3. What treatment would you give?

Paper 11 *Answers*

11

ANSWER 11.1

1. Ring sideroblast and a vacuolated promyelocyte
2. Pearson's syndrome
3. Bone marrow aspiration and mitochondrial DNA analysis

The combination of pancreatic and haematopoietic disorders suggests Pearson's syndrome. This is a rare condition associated with mitochondrial DNA rearrangements (large-scale deletions or duplications). It is sporadic and usually presents with sideroblastic anaemia that may be severe enough to cause hydrops fetalis. Neutrophils and platelets are affected in many patients and bone marrow often shows vacuolated precursors. Other classic features in early life include steatorrhoea, renal tubular and hepatic dysfunction and raised lactate concentrations in blood and CSF. Although diabetes mellitus occurs in about 30% of patients it is usually a later feature. Neurological features of Kearns–Sayre syndrome develop in patients surviving beyond the first 2 years. Bone marrow dysfunction tends to improve with time.

ANSWER 11.2

1. Constitutional
2. LHRH stimulation test – this should demonstrate a brief LH response as in puberty and would exclude central precocious puberty
3. Cranial imaging (CT or MRI)
4. LHRH analogues to suppress the hypothalamic–pituitary–gonadal function. This would be reserved for the cases where precocious puberty is likely to result in premature fusion of the bony epiphyses and short stature

The differential in this girl is whether or not she has a constitutional or cerebral cause for her precocious puberty. An isosexual pubertal progression with symmetrical ovarian maturation suggests activity of the hypothalamic–pituitary–gonadal axis.

The hypothalamic–pituitary–gonadal endocrine axis is established during fetal life. There are some transient surges of gonadotrophins and sex steroids

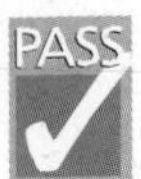

after birth and during infancy but these become suppressed during childhood. The mechanisms by which this occurs are poorly understood. A variety of cerebral insults (for example, trauma, tumours, infectious/inflammatory lesions, cysts and hydrocephalus) may provoke early puberty. In girls the LHRH pulse generator is more prone to early reactivation, and this accounts for most cases of precocious puberty. A central cause is more likely in boys or in girls who undergo puberty at a very early age. Treatment is given to those in whom the pubertal growth spurt would give rise to eventual shortened stature, for example very early puberty.

ANSWER 11.3

1. Benign intracranial hypertension
   Intracranial venous thrombosis
2. CT scan or MRI scan of head

This child has a number of features associated with raised intracranial pressure. The differential diagnosis is benign intracranial hypertension or intracranial venous thrombosis. Although immunosuppressed, it is unlikely that an infective central nervous system condition would produce the symptoms, signs and results described. She was given a lengthy course of corticosteroids to treat her renal condition. It is well recognised that prednisolone (and prednisolone withdrawal) can cause benign intracranial hypertension. Other causes of benign intracranial hypertension include infections (roseola infantum) haematological conditions (polycythaemia, haemolytic anaemia) and metabolic disorders (galactosaemia, hypophosphatasia). Treatment is either to reduce the volume of cerebrospinal fluid (CSF) with acetazolamide or frusemide or to remove CSF by lumbar puncture(s). Arterial and venous thromboses are a potentially fatal complication of nephrotic syndrome and relate to a number of factors including hypovolaemia, steroid use, increased platelet aggregation, loss of anti-thrombin III and raised levels of fibrinogen. They can occur in many locations including cerebral venous sinuses.

ANSWER 11.4

1. Non-alcoholic steatohepatitis (NASH) associated with obesity
2. Supervised and controlled dieting with weight loss
   Encouragement of active exercise

NASH is now commonly recognised in childhood and is associated with obesity and diabetes mellitus. The patients often present with abdominal pain, an asymptomatic hepatomegaly, transaminitis or an ultrasound suggestive of fatty infiltration of the liver. It is important to look for acanthosis nigricans, a cutaneous association that can be a clue to the underlying problem.

Hyperinsulinaemia, hypercholesterolaemia and hyperetriglyceridaemia can lead to excessive fatty infiltration of the liver. There is similar pathogenesis in Mauriac disease. The hepatic steatosis may not be entirely benign and

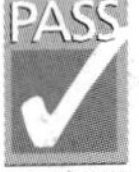

extensive fibrosis and cirrhosis has been reported on biopsy. Therefore dieting and weight loss should be actively pursued.

ANSWER 11.5

1. Zinc deficiency (acrodermatitis enteropathica)
2. Serum zinc level
3. Zinc supplementation

Zinc is an essential component of many enzymes and is involved in the synthesis of protein and RNA. Associations of zinc deficiency include poor growth (including intrauterine growth retardation), delayed wound healing, and in children hypogonadism and hepatosplenomegaly. Zinc accumulates in the fetus during the last trimester. Accretion rates in utero are far higher than the amounts used (if any) in parenteral nutrition solutions. Frank zinc deficiency in the preterm population is, however, relatively uncommon. Maternal milk may contain sufficient zinc to match in utero accretion rates in the first few months after preterm delivery but the amount present falls rapidly. In addition enteral zinc absorption is often poor until about 36 weeks' corrected gestation.

This infant's mother was vegetarian, which may have reduced the amount of zinc available in her breast milk as red meat may contain up to 10 times more zinc than vegetables and fruit. A serum zinc level was 0.1 μmol/l (normal range 5–15). After 2 weeks of zinc supplementation the rash had completely cleared and her serum zinc level had increased to 9.4 μmol/l. Breast milk zinc concentration at this time was 34.8 μmol/l (approximately 2.1 μg/ml). She was also noted to be iron deficient. At 1 year of age she was well, growing normally and making normal developmental progress.

Paper 12 *Questions*

12

QUESTION 12.1

A 13-month-old boy is referred with chestiness. He was born at term after a pregnancy complicated by maternal pneumonia, birthweight 3560 g. He was exclusively breast fed for 6 months. At the age of 5 months he had an episode clinically felt to be bronchiolitis. Since then he has had recurrent respiratory tract infections, more so during the winter months. His mother describes him as sounding 'rattly' but has not heard him wheeze on a regular basis. His symptoms are not worse at any particular time of the day or night and have not been helped by numerous courses of antibiotics or a variety of inhaled treatments, including ipratropium and steroids. A course of oral steroids produced no improvement. He has been fully immunised. There is a family history of eczema. His 3-year-old sister is well. On examination he looks well and is appropriately grown, with his height and weight on the 50th centile. He is not clubbed. There is moderate cervical lymphadenopathy, with enlarged, non-inflamed tonsils. Chest examination reveals a Harrison's sulcus with transmitted sounds from the upper airway; there is no audible wheeze.

Full blood count	normal
CXR	normal
Sweat test	normal
RAST to cow's milk	negative
Serum immunoglobulins & subclasses	normal
Serum tetanus antibody	< 0.05 IU/ml (normal > 0.1 IU/ml)
Serum *Haemophilus influenza* b antibody	1.02 μg/ml (normal > 1 IU/ml)
T and B lymphocyte subsets	normal
Neutrophil function	normal
pH probe	Fig. 12.1

1. Suggest a cause for the recurrent chesty episodes.
2. How would you manage him further? (List three)

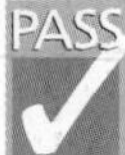

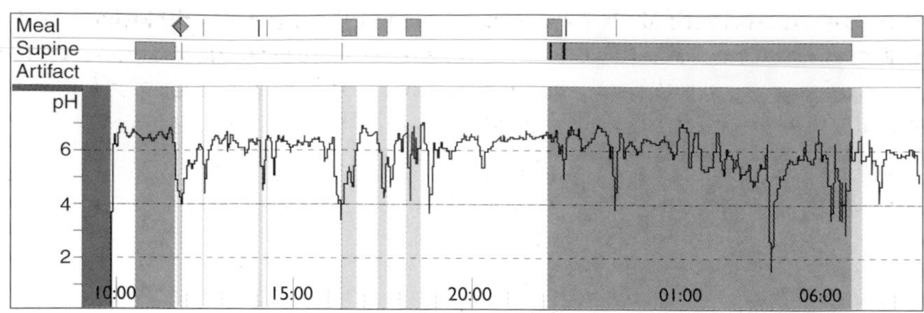

Fig. 12.1

QUESTION 12.2

A 12-year-old girl presents with a 36-hour history of fever and headache. Her parents report that she has been behaving strangely, with episodes of lip smacking. She lives with her parents and older sister. She is normally healthy, and her only previous admission to hospital was as an infant with a febrile convulsion. Her father has been taking antidepressants since he was made redundant 3 months ago. Her older sister has been caught shoplifting and is thought to be using 'recreational drugs'.

On examination she is febrile (38.1°C). She is clearly confused and disoriented in time and space. Her pulse rate is 88/min, blood pressure 110/70 mmHg. The remainder of the cardiovascular and respiratory examination is normal. Examination of cranial nerves, central and peripheral nervous system is unremarkable apart from the confusion. A lumbar puncture is performed. Initially bloodstained CSF is obtained but this clears as more CSF is obtained.

Haemoglobin	12.6 g/dl
White cell count	8.9×10^9/l
Neutrophils	1.8×10^9/l
Platelets	232×10^9/l
Serum urea & electrolytes	normal
Blood glucose	5.6 mmol/l
CSF microscopy	57 white cells/mm^3 (95% mononuclear), 510 red cells/mm^3
CSF protein	0.6 g/l
CSF glucose	3.6 mmol/l

1. What is the diagnosis?
2. List four investigations you would use to confirm this.
3. What treatment should be started?

QUESTION 12.3

A 2-week-old boy presented with diarrhoea. He was the only child of caucasian parents. His mother had recurrent urinary tract infections during pregnancy. He was breast fed and his mother was concerned that his stools were loose. On examination he looked well but a left loin mass was palpable. The baby was normotensive and no other abnormalities were noted. A normal stool was seen in his nappy. An abdominal ultrasound scan revealed a normal right kidney and a very large, abnormal left kidney. A micturating cystourethrogram demonstrated mild vesicoureteric reflux on the right with no reflux noted on the left. The patient's dimercaptosuccinic acid (DMSA) scan is shown (Fig. 12.2):

Serum sodium	136 mmol/l
Serum potassium	3.9 mmol/l
Serum urea	3.5 mmol/l
Serum creatinine	32 μmol/l
Serum calcium	2.45 mmol/l
Serum phosphate	1.90 mmol/l
Serum chloride	103 mmol/l
Serum bicarbonate	24 mmol/l
Urine dipstick	no blood, no protein

1. What is the most likely diagnosis?
2. What is its inheritance?

Fig. 12.2 ***Report:*** Split function: left 0%, right 100%

QUESTION 12.4

A 4-year-old boy is referred with a history of episodic persistent vomiting and chest infections often requiring hospital admission. He was a breech presentation and born by Caesarean section. He had feeding difficulties as an infant – particularly with a poor sucking reflex – and required supplemental nasogastric tube feeding for the first 6 months. Developmentally he sat unsupported at 11 months, and walked unaided at 24 months. His parents feel he is clumsy. His speech is slightly unclear but his comprehension is good. In the past, he was seen by the ophthalmologist for a corneal abrasion with delayed healing.

On examination, he is on the 25th centile for height and weight. He is not dysmorphic. He has a smooth tongue. He has cold peripheries but with all peripheral pulses palpable. His blood pressure lying is 80/62 mmHg and standing 66/40 mmHg. On auscultation, his heart sounds are normal but there are some coarse crepitations at the right base. Palpation of his abdomen is unremarkable. Fundoscopy is unremarkable. Knee and ankle reflexes are

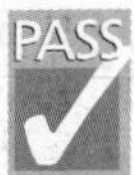

absent. Plantar reflexes are not attempted, as there is a fresh laceration of the sole of the right foot. His parents were unaware of this before consultation.

1. What is the diagnosis?
2. What two investigations will support this diagnosis?

QUESTION 12.5

A 6-week-old baby boy was referred to the clinic because the health visitor had reported that he had multiple bruises. There was a family history of von Willebrand's disease on the mother's side of the family and she was concerned that the baby might be affected. There were two older sisters, one of whom was in care following physical abuse from the mother's previous partner. The baby had been born after a pregnancy complicated by pregnancy-induced hypertension and had been delivered at 36 weeks for maternal reasons. There had been mild oozing from the cord and the cord had not separated until a week of age. In retrospect the parents thought that the baby had blue marks on the skin soon after birth. They were unsure whether new ones had developed but those that had been present had not disappeared. There had been no obvious trauma and no overt bleeding or the appearance of petechiae.

On examination the baby was well, alert and thriving. There were no petechiae, lymphadenopathy or hepatosplenomegaly. There was a small subconjunctival haemorrhage in the left eye. The skin had numerous bluish discoloured areas as illustrated below (Fig. 12.3).

1. What are the lesions?

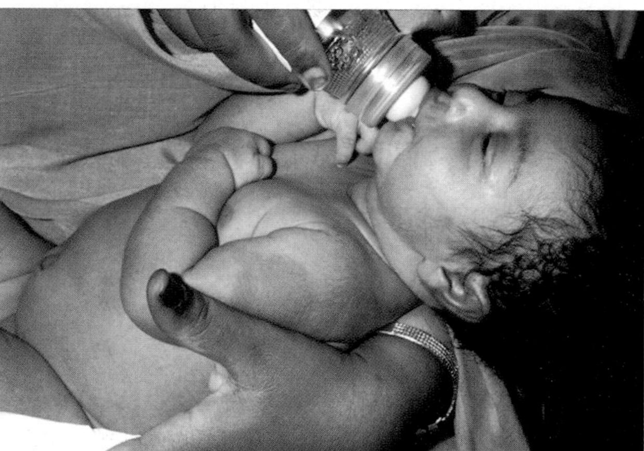

Fig. 12.3

Paper 12 *Answers*

12

ANSWER 12.1

1. Developmental 'immaturity' of immune system
2. Tetanus booster and recheck response
   Immunisation against *Pneumococcus* around 2 years of age
   Antibiotic prophylaxis during winter months

This boy's immune system is essentially normal, although it may be developmentally immature or undergoing a developmental pause. Antibiotic prophylaxis with co-trimoxazole may alleviate the problem, although it will not obliterate this completely. The response to protein antigens such as those in the Hib, tetanus or MMR vaccine evolve earlier than that to polysaccharide antigens such as those contained in the pneumococcal vaccine, and therefore whilst a tetanus booster is worthwhile pneumococcal vaccination is probably best delayed until about 2 years of age. The pH study shown is within normal limits: gastro-oesophageal reflux is assessed on the frequency and duration of episodes of pH < 4. The episodes here all demonstrate immediate recovery.

ANSWER 12.2

1. Viral (herpetic) meningoencephalitis
2. Herpes simplex PCR
   Viral titres
   Viral throat swabs
   Viral stool culture
3. High-dose intravenous acyclovir

The combination of the CSF result and the odd behaviour of this girl should point to the diagnosis of herpetic meningoencephalitis. Whilst the CSF was bloodstained the proportion of white cells to red cells is greater than 1 : 500, which would be seen in the absence of infection and with a traumatic tap. High-dose acyclovir therapy should be initiated pending the results of herpes simplex PCR results. Other less specific investigations include viral titres, viral throat swabs and viral stool culture. EEG changes do occur in Herpes simplex encephalitis; the classic unilateral paroxysmal latent epileptiform

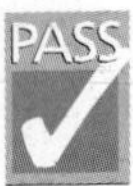

discharges are not pathognomonic but are characteristic. Nevertheless they are useful in localising the disease.

ANSWER 12.3

1. Unilateral multicystic dysplastic kidney
2. Sporadic

This baby has a loin mass, which is one of the more common postnatal presentations of a unilateral multicystic dysplastic kidney (MDK). The MDK is at the extreme end of the renal dysplasia spectrum and consists of many cysts of different sizes with no normal renal tissue present. It does not function at all. There is usually an associated atretic ureter and thus the kidney has no connection with the bladder. MDK is almost always a unilateral disorder: bilateral MDK usually results in fetal death. MDK is an uncommon, non-hereditary condition (although it is associated with syndromes such as Jeune's and Zellweger's) associated with hypertension, usually in later life, and very rarely with renal malignancy. Overall the prognosis is excellent. Abnormalities of the contralateral kidney are seen in approximately 50% of cases. Vesicoureteric reflux (as in this case) is the most common. Extrarenal abnormalities also occur and include tracheo-oesophageal fistula and ventricular septal defect.

The differential diagnosis includes a severe pelviureteric junction obstruction (PUJO), autosomal dominant and autosomal recessive polycystic kidney disease (ADPKD and ARPKD). However, in PUJO the calyces (which can be mistaken for cysts) communicate with the renal pelvis, some normal renal parenchyma will be visible on ultrasound scanning and uptake of isotope will be noted on the DMSA scan. Both ADPKD and ARPKD usually produce bilaterally large kidneys with bilateral activity seen on DMSA scanning. Also, in ADPKD normal renal tissue is noted between the cysts on ultrasound scanning and in ARPKD the cysts are usually much smaller than those seen in MDK.

ANSWER 12.4

1. Familial dysautonomia (Riley–Day syndrome)
2. Intradermal injection of histamine (absent flare – an axon reflex)
   Pilocarpine pupil reaction test (pupillary constriction because of denervation hypersensitivity)

Familial dysautonomia has both sensory and autonomic nervous system symptoms and should be completely diagnosable on clinical grounds. Although it is reported as an autosomal recessive disease in the Ashkenazi Jewish population, it can occur sporadically in non-Jewish children.

In the neonatal period hypotonia, hypothermia, poor feeding, and especially an absent suck reflex, are present. Motor incoordination becomes more apparent with age. Patients will have feeding difficulties, cyclical vomiting and recurrent pneumonia. Other symptoms include the failure to produce overflow tears, absent corneal reflexes, absent or diminished tendon reflexes, a labile blood pressure with postural hypotension, temperature instability and a relative indifference to pain. There are no specific diagnostic tests, though the above investigations will support the clinical diagnosis.

ANSWER 12.5

1. Mongolian blue spots

Mongolian blue spots typically occur over the sacroiliac region in 80% of babies of Asian or African origin. The blue or slate-grey colour of the macules results from deposition of the dermis of melanocytes, which are thought to have been arrested during migration to the epidermis from the neural crest. Most disappear by a year of age. Occasionally the lesions are multiple, as in this child. Malignant change does not occur.

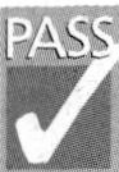

Paper 13 *Questions*

13

QUESTION 13.1

A set of male twins is born at 25 weeks' gestation, birthweights 750 g and 710 g. The smaller twin is noted to have hypospadias. They both require ventilation for respiratory distress syndrome and both develop pneumothoraces requiring formal chest drains. The larger twin requires ligation of a haemodynamically significant patent ductus arteriosus. By the age of 4 weeks they are both extubated in low concentrations of ambient oxygen. They have initial feed intolerance associated with sepsis, requiring periods of parenteral nutrition, but have both been receiving full enteral feeds (preterm formula) from the age of 3 weeks. The smaller twin has poor weight gain compared with his brother initially, although by the age of 6 weeks this is improving. Routine haematology and biochemistry has been stable. Bolus (gavage) feeds are introduced during the following week (corrected gestation 32 weeks). After 4 days the smaller twin becomes acutely unwell, with pallor and poor perfusion. His blood pressure is 75 systolic by Doppler. Physical examination is otherwise unremarkable. The following results are obtained from an infection screen:

Haemoglobin	12.9 g/dl
White cell count	5.8×10^9/l
Platelets	351×10^9/l
Serum sodium	175 mmol/l
Serum potassium	3.7 mmol/l
Serum urea	4.1 mmol/l
Serum creatinine	62 μmol/l
Blood glucose	4.2 mmol/l
Urine microscopy	no organisms, no cells
CSF microscopy	clear, colourless, no organisms seen
CSF glucose	3.1 mmol/l
CSF protein	normal
Chest radiograph	chronic lung disease
Abdominal radiograph	normal

1. List four investigations you would perform next.
2. Suggest a possible diagnosis.

QUESTION 13.2

An 11-month-old Asian girl is referred because of concerns by her health visitor. Only at 6 months did she start rolling over and she did not sit unsupported until 9 months. Now at 11 months she does not crawl or pull to a stand. She grasps objects and developed a pincer grasp at about 10 months. She started squealing and laughing at 7 months and babbling at 9 months. She only says 'dada' now. She was born at term, weighing 3210 g. There were no perinatal problems. She has been breast fed since birth, weaned at 4 months and is now reported to be taking a varied diet. Her weight followed 50th–75th centile from birth to 2 months. At the next measurement (7 months) it had dropped to just below the 3rd centile and now has deviated further below the 3rd centile. Her current length is on the 10th centile, her head circumference on the 75th centile.

She lives with her mother and two healthy siblings and is cared for about half the time by her maternal grandmother, who is supportive, caring and experienced. On examination there is bulbous non-tender enlargement of the wrists and palpable enlargement of the costochondral junctions. There are no deformities of her legs or thorax. She has relatively reduced muscle mass. Her anterior fontanelle is soft and widely open. Her muscle tone appears to be decreased generally but her reflexes are normal.

Full blood count	normal
Serum urea and electrolytes	normal
Serum bicarbonate	18 mmol/l
Serum calcium	1.75 mmol/l
Serum phosphate	0.8 mmol/l
Alkaline phosphatase	2257 IU (upper limit normal for age 850 IU)
Serum amino acid profile	non-specific increase in alanine and glycine
Urine amino acid profile	generalised aminoaciduria

1. What is happening with this girl's development?
2. What biochemical abnormality is present?
3. What is the diagnosis?
4. How does it cause this girl's developmental delay?
5. What treatment is needed?

QUESTION 13.3

A 15 year-old girl was diagnosed at 6 months of age with cystic fibrosis after failing to thrive. Until 12 months ago she had been generally well and had experienced only three lower respiratory tract infections requiring admission. Her symptoms were well controlled on oral antibiotics, vitamin and pancreatic supplements. She had thrived and been generally compliant with her medication and physiotherapy.

Over the last year her general condition had deteriorated. Her weight had gradually fallen and she needed three admissions with respiratory exacerbations. These were slow to resolve despite appropriate intravenous antibiotic therapy. Outpatient pulmonary function testing confirmed a reduction in her lung function. She had started a relationship with an older boyfriend, who her parents felt was 'involved in drugs'. Since that time she admitted to poor adherence to her treatments. On examination she had finger clubbing. Her weight was on the 0.4th centile and her height on the 25th. She had moderate facial acne. Examination of her respiratory system revealed a Harrison's sulcus, coarse left-sided basal crackles and widespread expiratory wheeze. Her abdomen was soft. Stool microscopy revealed a very small amount of fat.

Lung function testing:

Forced expiratory volume in 1 second (FEV_1)	50% of expected for height
Forced vital capacity (FVC)	80% of expected for height

1. Give two possible explanations for her recent deterioration?
2. List six further appropriate investigations?

QUESTION 13.4

A 2-year-old girl is referred because of concerns with poor weight gain. According to her mother, she eats extremely well but has excessive flatulence and passes very loose foul-smelling stools that are difficult to flush away. She was born at term with a birthweight on the 91st centile. She was admitted to hospital at 3 months of age with bronchiolitis and required ventilation for 5 days because of recurrent apnoeas. Since that time, she has been clinically well. She sat unsupported at 6 months and walked by herself at 14 months. On examination, her weight is on the 2nd centile. She has no finger clubbing. She has generalised dry skin without any excoriation. Her abdomen is distended and tympanic but with no organomegaly.

Haemoglobin	10.3 g/dl
White cell count	$6.3 \times 10^9/l$
Neutrophils	$3.1 \times 10^9/l$
Lymphocytes	$2.9 \times 10^9/l$
Platelets	$339 \times 10^9/l$
Blood film	moderate acanthocytosis, otherwise normal
Prothrombin time	17 s (control 11–15 s)
Activated partial thromboplastin time	33 s (control 24–35 s)
Serum alanine transaminase	normal
Serum albumin	39 g/l
IgA endomysial antibodies	negative
Sweat test	normal
Serum cholesterol levels	low
Serum triglyceride levels	low

1. What further investigations would you perform?
2. What is the diagnosis?
3. List three associated neurological problems.

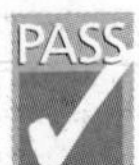

QUESTION 13.5

A 4-year-old Pakistani girl was brought to the clinic with a 6-month history of severe bruising. The bruises occurred episodically and without any obvious antecedent trauma. On questioning her mother thought that the child had always bruised easily but that it had got worse recently. The bruising had involved her trunk, limbs and face. She had never had epistaxis, haematuria or melaena. There was no joint involvement at any time. She had an older brother who was well. The parents were well and unrelated. Her father (who was not present in clinic) owned a general store where her mother helped out. Her mother was at a loss to explain the bruising. She could not think of any circumstances in which the child could have been physically abused, nor did she think it likely.

On examination the girl was well, friendly and appeared to relate well to her mother. Her height and weight were appropriate for her age. Examination was unremarkable except for a large fading bruise approximately 5 cm × 4 cm on the right flank. There were no purpura or lymphadenopathy and no splenomegaly.

Haemoglobin	10.8 g/dl
White cell count	$6.4 \times 10^9/l$
Platelets	$328 \times 10^9/l$
Blood film	normal
Coagulation screen	normal
Ristocetin platelet function	normal

Over the subsequent 3 months she developed further episodic bruising of a similar nature, once on her legs and once on her buttocks. Social services failed to find any evidence suggesting maltreatment and a skeletal survey was normal.

1. What is the most likely diagnosis?
2. How would you establish it?
3. How would you treat the condition?

Paper 13 *Answers*

13

ANSWER 13.1

1. Serum chloride
   Urine electrolytes
   Serum and urinary electrolytes in co-twin
   Milk sodium concentration
2. Malicious administration of salt

This infant's electrolyte picture does not fit a recognised pattern given the previous history of normal biochemistry. Urine electrolytes revealed high concentrations of sodium and the co-twin had a similar set of results. A high sodium concentration was found in the twins' formula: the mother subsequently admitted adding salt to their milk.

ANSWER 13.2

1. Delayed gross motor development
   Social, language and fine motor skills within normal limits
2. She has hypocalcaemia and secondary hypoparathyroidism
3. Nutritional rickets causing gross motor delay
4. There is phosphate depletion and decreased muscle strength in nutritional rickets
5. Vitamin D

Hypotonia and delayed motor development are commonly found in nutritional rickets. The mechanism is thought to be phosphate depletion and decreased muscle strength. If this is the case, motor skills improve promptly with vitamin D treatment. In nutritional rickets the transient manifestations of secondary hyperparathyroidism (plasma bicarbonate with a normal anion gap, generalised, non-specific aminoaciduria, low tubular reabsorption of phosphate) that are present in this infant might lead one to believe that this infant in fact has a congenital lesion of the proximal tubule leading to these findings of Fanconi syndrome. Measuring serum 1,25 hydroxyvitamin D concentration might add to the confusion; this is normal (or perhaps even high)

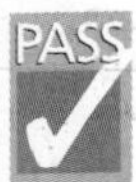

in nutritional rickets. Advice regarding vitamin supplementation during breast feeding is confusing, but in 'at risk' groups vitamin D therapy would prevent cases like this.

ANSWER 13.3

1. Non compliance
   Development of diabetes mellitus
2. Glycosylated haemoglobin
   Plasma glucose
   Urine dipstick testing for glucose
   Glucose tolerance test
   Detailed dietary history
   Chest radiograph

It may simply be that this adolescent is non-adherent with her various therapies and this has led to the worsening of her condition. A low stool fat content can simply reflect a low dietary fat intake. An alternative explanation is the development of type 1 diabetes. This occurs in 10% of patients over the age of 10 years and is often associated with a worsening in the patient's pulmonary function, weight loss, polyuria and polydipsia. Diabetic ketoacidosis is very rarely seen and the electrolyte disturbance is usually mild. It is usually readily amenable to treatment with dietary changes and small amounts of insulin.

ANSWER 13.4

1. Chylomicrons, VLDL, LDL and β-lipoprotein levels
   Electron microscopy of duodenal biopsy
   Vitamin A and E levels
2. Abetalipoproteinaemia
3. Ataxia, loss of vibration sense and position
   Atypical retinitis pigmentosa

This infant presents with a clinical picture of steatorrhoea and associated failure to thrive. Her dermatitis and coagulopathy reflect malabsorption of fat-soluble vitamins. The differential diagnosis should include other causes of fat malabsorption, for example coeliac disease and cystic fibrosis. The normal neutrophil count would exclude Shwachman's syndrome. The low plasma cholesterol and triglyceride levels and the presence of acanthocytes in the peripheral blood would suggest abetalipoproteinaemia. This autosomal recessive disease is due to a congenital deficiency of β-lipoprotein. Because of the absence of β-lipoprotein, chylomicrons cannot be formed and there is fat retention within intestinal epithelial cells. Neurological complications occur later in childhood. Treatment includes using medium-chain triglycerides to replace long-chain triglycerides in the diet and fat-soluble vitamin supplementation (particularly vitamin E).

ANSWER 13.5

1. Factor XIII deficiency
2. Measure factor XIII. Suspend a clot in 20% urea overnight
3. Give intravenous factor XIII (or cryoprecipitate) on a regular basis

The characteristic story of episodic pathological bruising with normal clotting studies, normal platelets and normal platelet function is characteristic of factor XIII deficiency. Factor XIII is responsible for making crosslinks between fibrin dimers, thus ensuring clot stabilisation. In its absence the clotting process occurs normally but the clot cannot be maintained and bleeding or bruising occurs, similar to that seen in haemophilia or von Willebrand's disease. Haemarthrosis is not a feature. Diagnosis is either by direct assay (preferable) or by demonstration that a clot cannot maintain itself in a hyperosmolar solution. Treatment (as in haemophilia) is with regular and acute episodic intravenous replacement. The condition is inherited as a recessive trait. This little girl subsequently had a brother who was also affected.

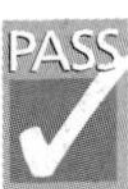

Paper 14 *Questions*

14

QUESTION 14.1

A male infant was born at 29 weeks' gestation to a single unsupported 17-year-old mother. He has severe hyaline membrane disease, requiring surfactant replacement therapy and high-frequency oscillation. He subsequently develops a significant shunt through a patent ductus arteriosus and is treated with indomethacin. This closes the duct but also results in an ileal perforation, necessitating laparotomy. He has a stormy postoperative course, requiring re-exploration of his abdomen.

He is slow to tolerate enteral feeds and requires parenteral nutrition for several weeks, which in turn causes a conjugated hyperbilirubinaemia with elevated liver enzymes. This gradually improves with the introduction of enteral nutrition. He also develops chronic lung disease as a consequence of his initial respiratory problems and requires a 6-week course of dexamethasone to wean him from the ventilator, in addition to diuretics. He was discharged home at 42 weeks' corrected gestation on oxygen and diuretics. He is generally difficult to handle and feed orally as a result of his prolonged period of intubation. He was admitted as an emergency 3 weeks later with apnoeas associated with a coryzal illness. A chest radiograph was performed (Fig. 14.1).

1. What does the radiograph show? List three features.
2. List four contributing factors for the findings.
3. What other diagnosis should be considered?

QUESTION 14.2

A 15-year-old girl is staying with relatives in the United Kingdom, having arrived from East Timor. She is normally fit and well but shortly after arrival in the country she became unwell and feverish. She was seen in the local GP's surgery 2 days ago, where she was diagnosed as having a urinary tract infection. She was started on nitrofurantoin. Her parents were told to bring her back if she did not improve. Since then she has become increasingly unwell, sleepy and lethargic. Her parents complained that her urine was very dark.

On examination she is ill, pale and lethargic. She is tachycardic with a pulse rate of 156/min. Her peripheries are cool and the capillary refill

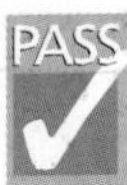

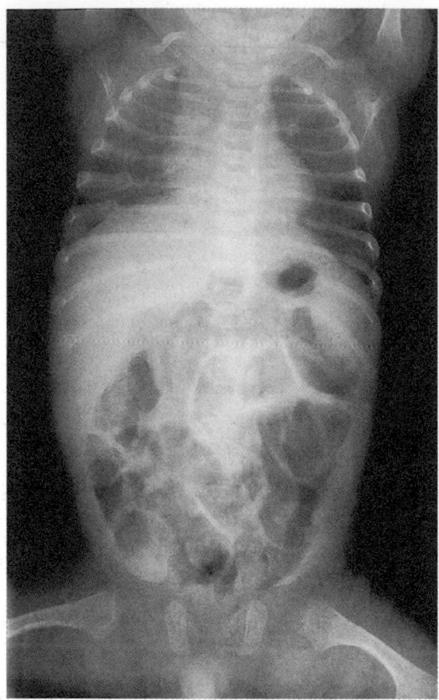

Fig. 14.1

>5 seconds. The respiratory rate was 44/min; her chest was clear on auscultation. Abdominal examination was unremarkable.

Urinalysis	blood +++
	urobilinogen +++
	protein ++
	no glucose
	no bilirubin

1. What immediate management should be undertaken?
2. List five urgent investigations you would perform.
3. What is your management after the initial admission period?
4. What is the most likely diagnosis?

QUESTION 14.3

A 9-month-old boy was reviewed because of abdominal pain and macroscopic haematuria. He had experienced intermittent pain and vomiting for 3 weeks, latterly associated with the passage of bloody urine into his nappy. He was born at 42 weeks' gestation and was small for dates. He had no neonatal problems. The referral letter from his GP noted that the family attended frequently for trivial illnesses but the boy had been generally well. His mother was very concerned about his appetite and regularly gave him herbal dietary supplements.

On examination he was well grown, with his height and weight both on the 50th centile. Although he had a systolic heart murmur, examination of the rest

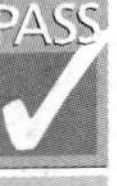

of his cardiovascular system was normal. Abdominal examination was unremarkable other than mild left-sided tenderness without guarding. Abdominal ultrasound scanning demonstrated marked bilateral renal medullary nephrocalcinosis and a single small stone in the distal left ureter.

Serum sodium	145 mmol/l
Serum potassium	4.7 mmol/l
Serum calcium	3.12 mmol/l
Serum albumin	40 g/l
Urinary oxalate/creatinine ratio	0.04 (normal <0.18)
Urinary calcium/creatinine ratio	1.52 (normal <0.8)

1. Give two differential diagnoses.
2. What additional investigations differentiate between the diagnoses?

QUESTION 14.4

An 11-month-old boy presents with fever and a productive cough. On the morning of admission he brought up fresh blood during a coughing bout on two occasions. He has suffered from a recurrent otitis externa and was admitted once previously with gastroenteritis. He is also under the care of the dermatology department for generalised eczema, which has partially responded to emollients and topical steroid cream. His 4-year-old brother has a peanut allergy and has been prescribed an Epipen. Otherwise there is no family history of note. On examination, his temperature is 38.2°C and his respiratory rate is 30/min. He has multi-coloured bruising over his back. A non-blanching purpuric rash is noted around his face and anterior neck. His eczema appears well controlled at present. On auscultation of his chest, course crepitations are heard at the right base. Splenomegaly is also noted.

Haemoglobin	$8.9 \times 10^9/l$
White cell count	$22.3 \times 10^9/l$
Neutrophils	$17.1 \times 10^9/l$
Lymphocytes	$4.1 \times 10^9/l$
Platelets	$25 \times 10^9/l$
Blood film	small platelets noted
Coombs test	positive
IgG	normal
IgA	increased
IgE	increased
IgM	reduced

1. What is the underlying diagnosis?
2. What is the long-term treatment?

QUESTION 14.5

A baby boy weighing 2955 g was born at 35 weeks to Pakistani parents. He needed no resuscitation and was transferred to the postnatal ward with his mother. At 48 hours of age he passed blood in his stool. On examination he

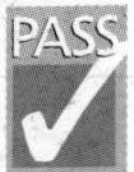

was noted to be jaundiced and a little drowsy. The liver was palpable 4 cm below the right costal margin. There was no splenomegaly and no other abdominal mass. Clinical examination revealed no other abnormal findings. A review of the history revealed that he had been breast feeding well until that morning, when he had seemed less interested. The parents were first cousins. There was no other significant family history.

Haemoglobin	12.3 g/dl
White cell count	19.6×10^9/l
Platelets	24×10^9/l
Prothrombin time	54 s (control 10–15 s)
Activated partial thromboplastin time	87 s (control 24–35 s)
Fibrinogen	1.2 g/l (normal 1.5–4.0 g/l)
Total serum bilirubin	309 μmol/l
Conjugated bilirubin	142 μmol/l
Serum aspartate transaminase	1256 IU/l (normal 5–50 IU/l)
Serum alkaline phosphatase	874 IU/l
Abdominal ultrasound	normal gall bladder and bile ducts. Liver parenchyma described as 'bright'

1. What other investigations would you perform?
2. What are the diagnostic possibilities?
3. What immediate treatment would you institute?

Paper 14 *Answers*

14

ANSWER 14.1

1. Fractures of three ribs on the right side
   Thin bone cortex
   Cupping/splaying of the rib ends
2. Prematurity
   Parenteral nutrition
   Steroid therapy
   Diuretic therapy
3. Non-accidental injury

This infant has had several factors operating during his time on the neonatal unit which will have contributed to metabolic bone disease. However, he has also been described as a 'difficult' infant and therefore the possibility of non-accidental injury must be considered.

ANSWER 14.2

1. Fluid resuscitation with 0.9% saline or colloid
2. Full blood count and blood film
   Serum urea and electrolytes
   Blood culture
   Urine culture
   Blood cross-match
3. Stop the nitrofurantoin
   Maintain hydration
   General cardiorespiratory supportive measures
   Treat symptomatic anaemia with cross-matched blood
4. Acute haemolysis precipitated by nitrofurantoin in a girl with glucose-6-phosphate dehydrogenase (G6PD) deficiency.

G6PD deficiency is the most common red cell enzyme defect. The incidence varies according to ethnic background, from rare in Caucasians to up to 25% in some Mediterranean people and in sub-tropical Asia and Papua New Guinea. Although the gene for G6PD is found on the X chromosome, the high

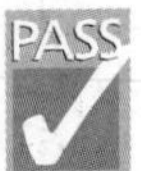

gene frequency in some populations means that homozygous females are not rare.

G6PD deficiency can present in a variety of ways. Most individuals with G6PD deficiency are asymptomatic. Neonatal jaundice is more common in boys of Chinese descent. Infections may precipitate haemolysis at any age. Haemolytic crises are of varying severity. The most fulminant is associated with ingestion of the fava bean (favism). Typical signs include darkening of the urine by blood and urobilinogen to a 'Coca-Cola' colour. The patient and her family will need to be given information regarding the diagnosis and implications for the affected child, particularly with respect to drugs and chemicals that can precipitate a haemolytic crisis. They should also be informed regarding the mode of inheritance and possible screening of male siblings.

ANSWER 14.3

1. William's syndrome
   Vitamin D toxicity
2. Plasma vitamin D level
   FISH analysis for the detection of elastin gene deletions

Nephrocalcinosis is uncommon in childhood and rare in the first year of life. During childhood it is usually restricted to the medulla and its causes include distal renal tubular acidosis, idiopathic hypercalciuria, idiopathic hypercalcaemia, vitamin D toxicity, William's syndrome, immobilisation, hypothyroidism and primary hyperoxaluria. Cortical nephrocalcinosis is usually seen only following renal cortical necrosis. In very early life nephrocalcinosis is usually caused either by the prolonged use of frusemide in the treatment of bronchopulmonary dysplasia or by primary hyperoxaluria.

The differential diagnosis in this case is between William's syndrome and vitamin D toxicity. This boy was post term, small for dates and had a heart murmur, all of which may be features of William's syndrome. Hypercalcaemia is rarely present after the first year but hypercalciuria persists. There is evidence that mutations in the elastin gene are responsible, at least in part, for the disorder. Vitamin D levels are normal. He was, however, given a 'herbal dietary supplement' which was discovered to contain large amounts of vitamin D.

ANSWER 14.4

1. Wiskott–Aldrich syndrome
2. Aggressive treatment of all infections
   Irradiated platelet transfusions for bleeding episodes
   Bone marrow transplantation

Wiskott–Aldrich syndrome is an X-linked recessive disorder characterised by chronic thrombocytopenia, eczema and immunodeficiency. The platelets are noted to be smaller in size. Bruising and petechiae are relatively common, but significant bleeding can also occur in up to 30% of patients. There may be an associated Coombs-positive haemolytic anaemia. The immunoglobulin profile shows high IgA and IgE with low levels of IgM. There are absent isohaemagglutinin antibodies, and low antibody titres to polysaccharide antigens such as haemophilus and pneumococcus. There is a progressive decrease in T-cell numbers and function during childhood.

Patients are susceptible to bacterial, viral and opportunistic infections and there is an increased incidence of autoimmune and lymphoproliferative disease. Conventional treatment includes prophylactic antibiotics, immunoglobulins and platelet transfusions. Splenectomy may improve the thrombocytopenia, though patients will be more prone to sepsis. Bone marrow transplantation has been successfully carried out.

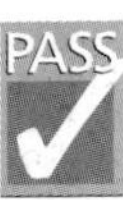

ANSWER 14.5

1. Septic screen, blood glucose, hepatitis and metabolic workup (including ammonia), serum ferritin
2. Septicaemia, liver disease with secondary bleeding diathesis (for example α-1-antitrypsin deficiency, ornithine transcarbamylase deficiency, galactosaemia)
3. Antibiotics, vitamin K, lactose-free/protein-free intake, antioxidant regimen

Sepsis should always be considered in any sick neonate. The association of hepatomegaly with bleeding raises the possibility of serious liver disease with a secondary bleeding diathesis (which might be fatal if left untreated). The parents' first-cousin relationship increases the likelihood of homozygous inheritance of a recessive condition; male gender raises the possibility of ornithine transcarbamylase deficiency. The prolonged PT and PTT could be a simple result of Vitamin K deficiency, although this is unlikely given the other clinical abnormalities and transaminitis. Haemorrhagic disease secondary to vitamin K deficiency is more likely to occur in infants with liver disease and in those who are breast fed (though it often presents slightly later), so first-aid treatment with parenteral vitamin K is essential. The timing is right for the onset of problems associated with an inability to catabolise protein so cessation of protein input is critical until a diagnosis has been made or refuted. Galactosaemia may present with bleeding problems associated with liver dysfuntion or Gram-negative septicaemia; antibiotic therapy and avoidance of lactose are important until an enzymatic assay has provided an answer. Alpha-1-antitrypsin deficiency has been reported to present in this way. Cystic fibrosis is unlikely given the racial background and the absence of other features. The echogenic appearance of the liver might be non-specific but it is characteristic when there is increased deposition of iron.

The baby became progressively more unwell in spite of supportive treatment and died as transfer to a transplant centre was being arranged. The only abnormal metabolic finding was an extremely high serum ferritin. This is highly suggestive of congenital iron storage disease, neonatal haemochromatosis (a recessively inherited condition). Post-mortem liver specimens confirmed the presence of large quantities of stainable iron.

Paper 15
Questions

15

QUESTION 15.1

A male infant is born at 34 weeks' gestation, birthweight 1400 g. Bilateral fetal renal pelvis dilatation (4 mm AP diameter) had been seen on ultrasound at 20 weeks and this was unchanged on a postnatal scan. He is in good condition at birth but develops respiratory distress within the first hour, needing CPAP support. He deteriorates over the next 12 hours and is therefore intubated, ventilated and given surfactant. His respiratory status improves slowly and on the fifth day he develops a significant patent ductus arteriosus, for which he receives a 3-day course of indomethacin. His cranial ultrasound is normal. On day 10 his electrolytes reveal hyponatraemia (121 mmol/l), having been normal 48 hours previously. He is by now receiving about 30% of his fluids enterally (preterm formula). He is given appropriate sodium replacement therapy over 24 hours and the following results are obtained. He passes approximately 50 ml of urine over this period. Biochemical results are as follows:

Table 15.1

	Na^+ (mmol/l)	*K^+ (mmol/l)*	*Urea (mmol/l)*	*Creatinine (μmol/l)*
Serum	118	4.7	2.6	49
Urinary	81	12.0	20.0	400

Urine microscopy   no cells or organisms seen

At this stage he becomes unwell, with a clinical picture of septicaemia associated with hypotension, a raised circulating white blood count and thrombocytopenia. He is commenced on broad-spectrum antibiotics and inotropic support pending culture results.

1. What do these results suggest as the reason for the hyponatraemia?
2. What may this be due to?
3. Suggest two further investigations.
4. What additional treatment would you consider?

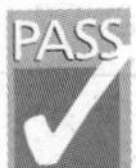

QUESTION 15.2

A 14-month-old boy presents to the local Accident and Emergency department with swelling of his head. Five days previously he had hit his head following a fall at nursery. This did not stop him playing and there was no reported loss of consciousness. Swelling began to be visible on the left side of his head. His mother took him to his GP, who reports seeing a firm swelling from the left occiput to left anterior parietal area. Two days later he was taken back to his GP with further swelling, now enlarged to involve the entire left scalp and extending to periorbital soft tissue. On examination he is well grown and afebrile. There is swelling involving the entire left scalp and extending to periorbital soft tissue. The left eye appears to be proptosed.

Haemoglobin	8.9 g/dl
White cell count	$5.4 \times 10^9/l$
Platelets	$505 \times 10^9/l$
Prothrombin time	13.9 s (normal 11–15 s)
Activated partial thromboplastin time	46 s (normal 24–35 s)
Fibrinogen	4.6 g/l (normal 1.5–4.0 g/l)

1. What single test will make the diagnosis in this boy?
2. What is the pathology behind the head and orbital swelling?
3. How should this boy be managed?

QUESTION 15.3

A 7-year-old boy was reviewed because of problems at school. Despite having some friends in his class, he was being teased because of his monotonous high-pitched voice. His teacher also noted that he was unable to play football with his classmates. Although he had difficulty in kicking the ball, his main problem was that he did not appear to understand the rules. He was assessed by the school to be of normal intelligence. From birth he was described as a very content baby, satisfied to lie alone in his cot for hours. There were no neonatal problems. He achieved normal developmental milestones but he initially had immature speech. His speech rapidly became age appropriate and was then considered by his parents to be advanced. His sister had cerebral gigantism.

On examination there were no significant clinical abnormalities other than gross motor incoordination. He was not dysmorphic and there was no obvious visual or hearing loss. His blood pressure was 105 mmHg systolic.

1. What is the diagnosis?
2. Give one investigation that should be performed.

QUESTION 15.4

A 14-year-old girl presents with a 3-month history of anorexia and weight loss. She complains of regular nausea and vomits after any attempt at eating solid foods. She has been sleeping very poorly and has been complaining of intermittent abdominal pain. She has been opening her bowels twice a day and there has been no obvious blood. She had her menarche at 11 years old but has no period for 10 months. Her mother feels that her daughter has lost approximately 5 kg in the last 2 months. Last year she had been bullied at school, but this has been sorted out as far as her mother is aware. In the family history her father has been treated for irritable bowel disease and her maternal grandmother has hypothyroidism. On examination, her weight is on the 3rd centile and her height on the 9th centile. She is pale with angular stomatitis. She also has moderate dental caries. Palpation of her abdomen is unremarkable.

Haemoglobin	8.9 g/dl
MCV	66.1 fl
White cell count	$5.3 \times 10^9/l$
Platelets	$773 \times 10^9/l$
ESR	21 mm/h
Serum protein	58 g/l
Serum albumin	33 g/l
T_4	normal
TSH	increased

1. What is the diagnosis?
2. What three further investigations would you do?
3. What is the present management of this problem?

QUESTION 15.5

A 10-year-old girl was admitted to hospital with fever, a rash, signs of meningeal irritation and a facial palsy. She had had asthma and eczema since early childhood but only occasionally had to use medication. She had last been well when the family went on holiday for 3 weeks, camping in Germany. Shortly after they returned she developed a painful and itchy area of erythema around an old insect bite, associated with a mild headache and non-specific malaise. The erythema spread over the next week but improved slowly when it was treated with 1% hydrocortisone. Three weeks later she again developed a rash, this time widespread. Two days before admission she had woken to find that she was unable to move the left side of her face or close her left eye. On the morning of admission she had developed a fever, headache, photophobia and neck stiffness.

On examination she was conscious but unwell and toxic with a fever of 39°C. Her conjunctivae were injected, Kernig's sign was positive and she had neck stiffness. There was a lower motor neurone facial palsy on the left. There was a widely disseminated macular red rash with lesions measuring from 0.5 to 1 cm across. The remainder of the clinical examination was normal.

Haemoglobin	12.3 g/dl
White cell count	$5.7 \times 10^9/l$
Neutrophils	$1.9 \times 10^9/l$
Platelets	$189 \times 10^9/l$
C-reactive protein	124 mg/l

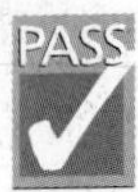

Blood glucose	5.7 mmol/l
CSF microscopy	145 white cells (100% lymphocytes)/mm^3
CSF glucose	4.5 mmol/l
CSF protein	1.2 g/l

1. What is the likely cause of this girl's illness?

Paper 15 *Answers*

15

ANSWER 15.1

1. Renal loss of sodium
2. Adrenal steroid insufficiency
3. Serum 17-hydroxyprogesterone
   Urine steroid profile
4. Intravenous hydrocortisone

This child has a salt-losing state (fractional excretion of sodium 8.4%), which does not appear related to either an intracranial event or to the administration of indomethacin. The renal pelvis dilatation and the serum creatinine are within normal limits, and therefore a primarily renal cause for the hyponatraemia is unlikely. It is essential to exclude congenital adrenal hypoplasia but the child's clinical condition warrants treatment with hydrocortisone before the results are available. The urine steroid profile will help determine the precise abnormality.

ANSWER 15.2

1. Measurement of coagulation factors VIII and IX.
2. There is a subgaleal haematoma extending into the orbit causing proptosis and compression of the globe. His coagulation study suggests previously unrecognised haemophilia (large masses of blood like this one in haemophilia sufferers are called pseudotumours)
3. There should be initial correction of the clotting factor deficiency and urgent surgical decompression of the orbit to protect vision

Haemophilic pseudotumour is a rare complication of haemophilia (pseudotumour occurs in both factor VIII and factor IX deficiencies). It can be found in 1–2% of patients with severe haemophilia. Its principal sites of occurrence are the long bones and the pelvis. Whilst decompression of the orbit needs to be performed urgently, recognition of the coagulation disorder before surgery, with subsequent correction using the appropriate clotting factor, is essential. Presentation and clinical severity of both haemophilia A and B depend on the level of clotting factors present.

ANSWER 15.3

1. Asperger's syndrome
2. X-chromosome analysis for fragile sites

This boy has many of the features of Asperger's syndrome. He appears to be very articulate as he uses parroted phrases that he has overheard. He also has peculiar voice characteristics. These are two of the most common associated speech and language problems. He also has motor clumsiness, which is considered to be a diagnostic criterion. An all-absorbing narrow interest is another diagnostic feature and, although not noted in the question, this boy developed a very keen interest in aeroplanes at the age of 5 years and became knowledgeable to a striking degree. He had no other interests.

Asperger's syndrome is further characterised by non-verbal communication problems, the imposition of routines and severe impairment in reciprocal social interaction. This boy was able to take part in some transient friendships, although these were very abnormal. By contrast, children with autism are more severely affected. Autism is characterised by a severe pervasive lack of responsiveness to all other people, a markedly restricted repertoire of activities and interests and a severe impairment in imaginative activity and verbal/non-verbal communication.

The fragile X syndrome can share some features of Asperger's syndrome. It has been recommended that all children diagnosed with Asperger's syndrome have chromosomal analysis. Despite the similarities, individuals with fragile X usually have global developmental delay; dysmorphic features and, in boys, increased testicular size.

ANSWER 15.4

1. Crohn's disease and sick euthyroid syndrome
2. Radio-isotope labelled white cell scan
   Endoscopy and colonoscopy with multiple biopsies
   Contrast follow-through
3. Polymeric or elemental diet
   On-going nutritional support
   Iron supplementation
   5-aminosalicyclic acid as maintenance treatment

Crohn's disease can often mimic anorexia nervosa or non-specific abdominal pain. Anorexia, weight loss, growth failure are more likely in Crohn's disease where as bloody diarrhoea is more prominent in ulcerative colitis. Children with chronic debilitating illnesses can suffer from sick euthyroid syndrome, which will respond to treating the primary illness. A polymeric diet is now the standard treatment for Crohn's disease of the small bowel or right-sided colon disease and is more acceptable to patients than the unwanted side-effects of steroids. Both upper and lower endoscopy is advocated for diagnostic purposes, as sometimes colonic biopsies can be non-specific.

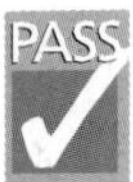

ANSWER 15.5

1. Lyme disease

The association of two episodes of an irritant rash with a facial palsy, systemic symptoms and (probable) aseptic meningitis following a visit to the USA would make Lyme disease the most likely diagnosis. In the USA the infection is endemic in New England and the eastern Pacific coast. Most cases in Europe occur in Scandinavia or central Europe. It is acquired when a bite is received from an insect carrying the spirochaete *Borrelia burgdorferi*. Classical signs are the appearance of an expanding irritant macular rash (erythema migrans) within 2–3 weeks of the bite, a secondary disseminated phase associated with a recurrence of the rash, fever, myalgia and headache and (sometimes) a radiculoneuritis or aseptic meningitis. Facial palsy is more common in children. Diagnosis is on clinical grounds. Treatment is with doxycycline, amoxicillin or ceftriaxone.

Paper 16 *Questions*

16

QUESTION 16.1

A 12-year-old boy is referred with difficult to control asthma. He was born at term after an uneventful pregnancy and did not require admission to the neonatal unit. He was well up to the age of 8 months, when he developed a productive cough, which resolved after several weeks. He had remained 'chesty' since that time, sometimes producing sputum. He had also had recurrent catarrhal symptoms from the age of 3 years. At the age of 6 years he had a 3-month bout of almost incessant coughing. Subsequently he regularly produced green sputum, through the winter months in particular, occasionally associated with wheeze. This generally responded to a combination of antibiotics and inhaled steroids and bronchodilators. He had been fully immunised. His symptoms were becoming more frequent, especially when he participated in any sport at school. His parents had recently separated and her mother felt that his schoolwork had suffered as a result. A maternal grandfather had been treated for tuberculosis in the past.

On examination his height was on the 50th centile and his weight on the 10th. He had a productive-sounding cough but appeared otherwise well. There was no clubbing. He had a mildly hyperinflated chest with coarse crackles at the left base and scattered wheeze on forced expiration. A chest radiograph was performed (Fig. 16.1).

1. What does the radiograph show?
2. List six other investigations you would perform.
3. What is the likely cause of the problem?
4. What are the treatment options?

QUESTION 16.2

A 13-year-old, previously healthy girl is referred through the educational psychology service with a 2-year history of declining academic performance and decreasing cognitive ability. She is also having increasing difficulty with motor activities and finds participation in sports is becoming more difficult. Her mother reports that her behaviour is becoming somewhat more erratic. Past medical history is unremarkable. Family history reveals that her parents

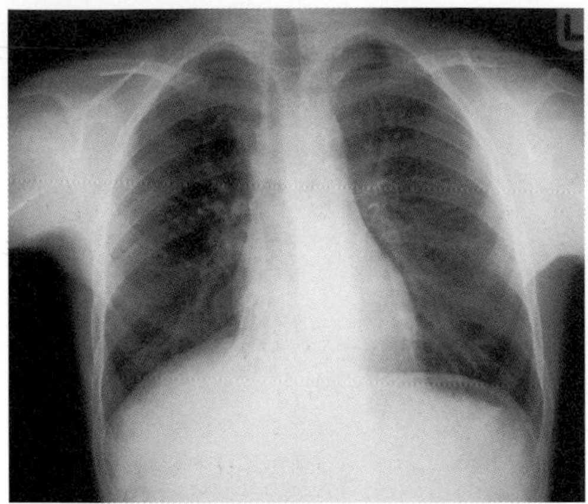

Fig. 16.1

and two siblings are in good general health. She lives with her mother and siblings. Her father left the household after a series of affairs and subsequent divorce.

On examination she is normotensive (122/76 mmHg) and with a pulse rate of 88/min. She is thin, with a weight of 37 kg. Examination of the chest, heart and abdomen failed to reveal abnormalities. Neurological examination demonstrated pupils that were equal, round and reactive to light and accommodation. She had difficulty with smooth pursuit and lateral saccades, and showed an overshooting and nystagmus on rapid movements of the eyes. Facial movements were symmetrical and facial sensation was intact. Hearing and vision were grossly unimpaired. Motor examination showed minimal weakness, but no atrophy or fasciculations were noted. Reflexes were symmetrical with no pathological reflexes and sensation was intact. She was noted to have abnormalities of co-ordination as well as with her gait.

Full blood count	normal
ESR	normal
Serum urea & electrolytes	normal
Liver function tests	normal
Caeruloplasmin	2.1 μmol/l (normal 1.3–2.7 μmol/l)
ASO titre	1: 800

1. What is the likely diagnosis in this girl?
2. What is the mode of inheritance?

QUESTION 16.3

A 3-year-old girl was referred with a sudden onset of stroke and coma. She had been well until a week before, when she and the rest of her family had gastroenteritis. She had very severe diarrhoea and abdominal pain, but this settled after a few days. Subsequently she began to vomit again and was noticeably quiet and pale. She then became restless and irritable and developed a tremor. Later that day she became weak on the left side and ultimately comatose. There was no significant past medical or family history.

On admission she was pale and had some bleeding from her buccal membrane. There were a number of small bruises over her legs. She had a dense left hemiplegia and a Children's Coma Scale score of 5. Her blood pressure was 90/70 mmHg. She had Kussmaul respirations and a smell of ketones on her breath.

Serum sodium	131 mmol/l
Serum potassium	7.5 mmol/l
Serum bicarbonate	10 mmol/l
Serum urea	45.7 mmol/l
Blood glucose	67 mmol/l
Serum amylase	850 IU/l (normal 75–300 IU/l)
Haemoglobin	8.5 g/dl
White blood count	$33.2 \times 10^9/l$ (neutrophils 75%)
Platelets	$25 \times 10^9/l$

1. What is the likely underlying diagnosis?
2. What two complications does this girl have?
3. Suggest four further investigations to support the diagnosis.

QUESTION 16.4

A 2-week-old girl is referred with a history of loose and bloody stools. She was born at term with a birthweight of 3800 g. She has been exclusively breast fed. Her mother, a chocolate addict, feels that she has been an unsettled baby since birth and has always passed loose stools. She possets regularly although her mother has not noticed any blood or bile. The baby has had a sticky umbilicus which responded to treatment with flucloxacillin. Her parents are fit and well. They also have a 4-year-old son, who has been admitted twice to hospital with acute exacerbations of asthma. On examination she is afebrile. Her weight is 4050 g and she is rather unsettled. She has seborrhoeic dermatitis, and generalised dry skin. Oral thrush is noted, though her perineum and anal margin appear normal. Palpation of the abdomen is unremarkable. Her nappy contains a poorly formed and bloody stool.

Haemoglobin	12.8 g/dl
White cell count	$13.0 \times 10^9/l$
Neutrophils	$6.2 \times 10^9/l$
Lymphocytes	$4.3 \times 10^9/l$
Basophils	$0.2 \times 10^9/l$
Eosinophils	$2.3 \times 10^9/l$
Platelets	$445 \times 10^9/l$
Stool culture	negative

1. What is the diagnosis?
2. List five further investigations.
3. What is the management?

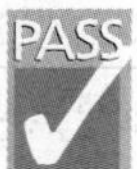

QUESTION 16.5

The paediatrician was asked to see a baby at 45 hours of age on the postnatal ward because of a suspicion of fitting. The baby had been born to a 40-year-old mother who had had an assisted conception. The pregnancy had been uneventful until 39 weeks' gestation, when the mother developed a urinary tract infection that was treated with antibiotics. Labour had occurred spontaneously at 41 weeks and the baby was delivered by rotational forceps for persistent occipitoposterior position. Apgar scores had been 7 at 1 minute and 9 at 5 minutes and the baby had required no resuscitation. He had been apparently well during the preceding 48 hours and had been breast feeding normally.

On examination he was noted to have clonic twitching of the right side of the face, right arm and right leg, which became generalised over a period of 2 or 3 minutes. The movements stopped spontaneously after 5 minutes and the baby started to cry. He was put to the breast and fed normally. Clinical examination at that time revealed no significant abnormalities.

CSF microscopy	5 white cells/mm^3, 20 red cells/mm^3
CSF protein	1.1 g/l
CSF glucose	3.5 mmol/l
Cranial ultrasound	Fig. 16.2

The baby was given a loading dose of phenobarbital intravenously and, apart from one brief similar episode 12 hours later, made an uneventful recovery and was discharged home at 1 week of age.

1. What is the most likely pathology underlying the clinical presentation?
2. What is shown on the cranial ultrasound scan?
3. What is the outlook for this boy's neurodevelopmental progress?

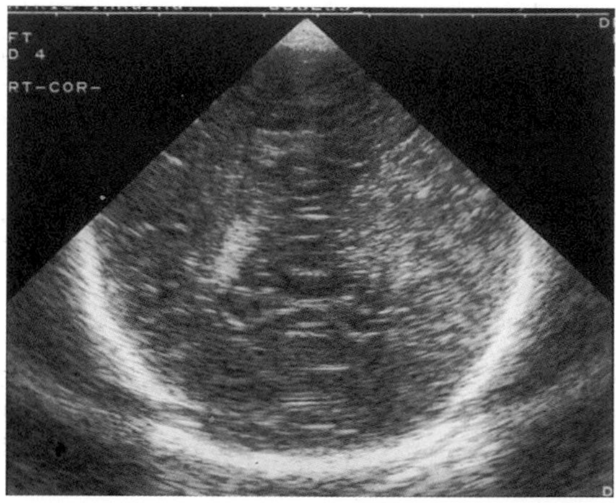

Fig. 16.2

Paper 16 *Answers*

16

ANSWER 16.1

1. Right lower lobe bronchiectasis
2. Sweat test
   Full blood count and differential
   Serum immunoglobulins and IgG subclasses
   Specific antibody titres
   High-resolution chest CT scan
   Cilial studies
3. Bronchiectasis following pertussis-like illness or severe adenovirus infection
4. Regular physiotherapy/antibiotics
   Lobectomy

This boy's problems are likely to be secondary to a pertussis-like illness, as suggested by the history (even though he was immunised). It is important to determine whether the problem is localised to one area of the lung or whether it results from a generalised problem, hence the need for immunological investigations and cilial function studies. Abnormalities of cilial function are associated with dextrocardia in only about 50% of cases. In the absence of other pathology, high-resolution CT scanning (Fig. 16.3) will help determine whether the affected area is amenable to surgical removal.

ANSWER 16.2

1. Juvenile-onset Huntington's disease (Westphal variant)
2. Autosomal dominant

Huntington's disease (HD) is an autosomal dominant neurodegenerative disorder characterised by motor, cognitive and behavioural dysfunction. The hallmark of the disorder is involuntary choreiform and athetotic movements; hence it is also known as Huntington's chorea. Approximately 10% of all patients with Huntington's disease present before the age of 20 years.

In 1993, a novel gene on the short arm of chromosome 4 containing a polymorphic CAG trinucleotide repeat was cloned and HD patients were

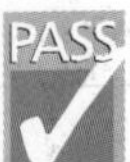

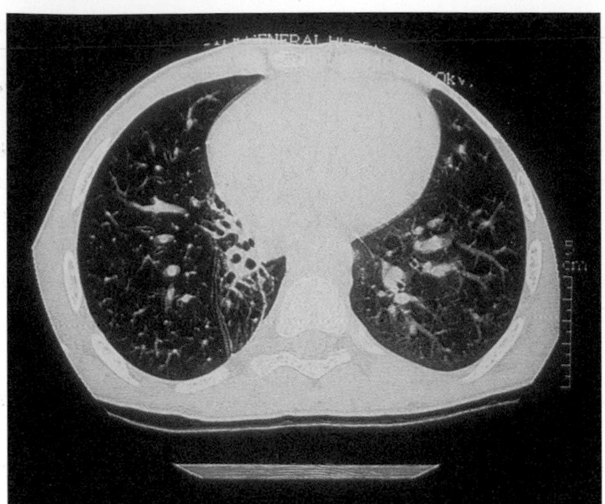

Fig. 16.3

found to have expansions of this CAG repeat. Approximately 99% of patients with a clinical diagnosis of Huntington's disease have an expanded allele, with 36 or more CAG repeats. Normal individuals have up to 35 CAG repeats, while affected HD patients almost always have an allele with 40 or more CAG repeats. Individuals with 36–39 repeats show 'reduced penetrance', meaning that only some will show clinical symptoms. An interesting genetic feature of HD is anticipation, which may be defined as worsening disease severity in successive generations. Research has shown that there is a correlation between the length of the CAG repeat and the age of onset and age of death in HD. Further expansion of the CAG repeat occurs much more frequently with paternal transmission than maternal transmission of the CAG repeat.

Juvenile HD patients typically do not present with chorea, but instead with rigidity or seizures. With progression of disease, classic uncontrolled, choreoathetotic movements do develop. Behavioural, cognitive or psychiatric difficulties are prominent. Although degeneration and atrophy in the caudate and putamen are seen in juvenile HD patients as in adult-onset HD patients, a more widespread pattern of neurodegeneration is usually seen both radiologically and neuropathologically. Neuronal loss in the Purkinje and granule cells of the cerebellum is common, as is atrophy of the dentate nucleus, globus pallidus, hippocampus and neocortex.

ANSWER 16.3

1. Diarrhoea-associated (D+) haemolytic uraemic syndrome
2. Severe neurological involvement
   Pancreatic involvement
3. Blood film
   Plasma creatinine
   Stool for VTEC 0157
   VTEC 0157 serology

This girl has severe diarrhoea-associated haemolytic uraemic syndrome with acute renal failure and significant extrarenal involvement. She has severe central nervous system involvement. The endothelial cell injury that occurs in the renal vessels is also seen in the cerebral vasculature in these individuals. The incidence of stroke and coma in diarrhoea-associated haemolytic uraemic syndrome are both reported to be 5%. The incidence of chronic neurological sequelae is also 5%. Other features indicative of severe central nervous system disturbance include seizures, dystonic posturing and cortical blindness. Minor central nervous system dysfunction such as somnolence and irritability are seen in most patients. Pancreatic involvement is seen in less than 10% of cases and can range from minor glucose intolerance to the picture of diabetic ketoacidosis illustrated. Clearly, features such as thrombocytopenia, anaemia, acute renal failure and focal neurological signs make diabetic ketoacidosis highly unlikely as the sole diagnosis in this case. Many other extrarenal sites may be involved in diarrhoea-associated haemolytic uraemic syndrome, such as the liver, lung, heart and gallbladder.

ANSWER 16.4

1. Cows' milk protein intolerance (CMPI)
2. Serum IgE levels
   RAST test to cows' milk protein
   Colonoscopy with biopsies
   Stool for *Clostridium difficile* culture
   Stool for *Clostridium difficile* toxin
3. Advise mother to go on to a cows' milk protein exclusion diet
   Active encouragement to continue breast feeding

Cows' milk protein intolerance can present even in breast-fed infants, as there is excretion of the protein in maternal breast milk that is then ingested by the infant. Gastro-oesphageal reflux, colic and a frank colitis are possible gastrointestinal presentations. A strong family history of atopy and an eosinophilia on the blood film would support this. In the differential diagnosis, although antibiotic-induced colitis and candidiasis were considered, it is the causal relationship to the symptoms that makes CMPI the most likely.

ANSWER 16.5

1. Stroke
2. Abnormal echodensity in left parietal region
3. Probable hemiplegia ± fits

Neonatal stroke occurs in 0.2/1000 term infants and is the most common cause of seizures apart from perinatal asphyxia. The aetiology is uncertain but it is thought to result from an embolus into the middle cerebral artery territory from either the placental bed or the ductus venosus. The left side is affected most frequently. Cortical lesions are more commonly associated with neonatal fits. The presentation is typically at 24–48 hours of age in a

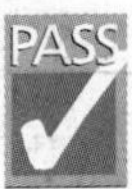

previously well baby. Ultrasound imaging may be normal early on but typically shows an abnormal focal echodensity in the middle cerebral artery territory. The investigation of choice is MRI at 1–2 weeks of age. Most babies recover quickly from the initial episode. Some 50% continue to have focal fits in childhood and 50–75% have a focal neurological defect, usually a hemiparesis, or more subtle signs.

Paper 17 *Questions*

17

QUESTION 17.1

A male infant is born at term by ventouse delivery for failure to progress after an uneventful pregnancy. Membranes were ruptured 22 hours before delivery. He requires minimal resuscitation and is transferred to the postnatal ward. At 36 hours of age he is noted to be pyrexial, 37.4°C, feeding poorly and tachypnoeic. He is transferred to the neonatal unit where his oxygen saturation is 91% in air. A full blood count and blood cultures are taken and he is commenced on intravenous antibiotics.

Haemoglobin	17.5 g/dl
White cell count	$17.1 \times 10^9/l$
Platelets	$92 \times 10^9/l$
Capillary pH	7.39
Capillary pCO_2	4.3 kPa
Capillary pO_2	6.1 kPa
Base deficit	–2.3 mmol/l

He initially requires up to 35% ambient oxygen to maintain oxygen saturations but is in air 24 hours after admission. A further 24 hours later he again deteriorates, with pallor, tachypnoea and increasing oxygen requirements. He subsequently requires intubation and ventilation. Blood cultures from admission are negative. A chest radiograph is performed (Fig. 17.1).

1. List four abnormal features on the chest radiograph.
2. Suggest the most likely diagnosis.

QUESTION 17.2

A 9-year-old boy is referred by his GP with a history of haemoptysis, dyspnoea and fever. This began with a productive cough 3 days earlier, for which he was prescribed amoxicillin. He continued to produce brown–green sputum, with obvious blood streaks becoming apparent. He had had a similar episode of haemoptysis 12 months previously and had recently been noted to wheeze. He had been commenced on salbutamol and beclomethasone inhalers without much improvement. On examination he looked pale.

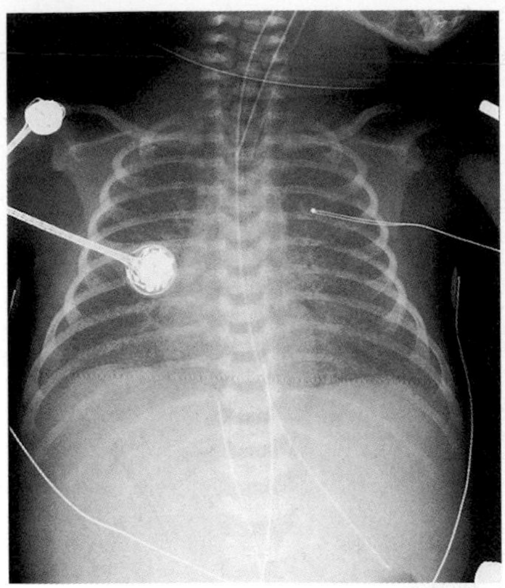

Fig. 17.1

Oxygen saturations in air were 84%. He was tachypnoeic (rate 44/min) and tachycardic (146/min). Axillary temperature was 38°C. Auscultation of his chest revealed widespread inspiratory crepitations and expiratory wheezes.

Haemoglobin	6.7 g/dl
White cell count	8.4×10^9/l
Platelets	141×10^9/l
MCV	68 fl
MCHC	24 g/dl
Blood culture	negative
Sputum culture	negative
Chest radiograph	Widespread diffuse bilateral micronodular shadowing with atelectasis in the right middle and lower lobes. Bilateral hilar lymphadenopathy

1. What is the most likely diagnosis?
2. What one confirmatory investigation would you consider in this boy?
3. How would you manage his symptoms?

QUESTION 17.3

A 14-year-old boy presented with genu valgum. His mother was an orthopaedic nurse. At 9 years of age he fractured his left distal ulna and radius following a fall. At age 10 he fractured his right tibia playing football; 6 months later his knock-knees were noticed. He was reviewed and the deformity was considered to relate to poor setting of his tibial fracture. The degree of deformity worsened over the following 3 years and he became unable to run or play football.

As a baby he was breast fed and fed voraciously. He has always wanted large amounts of fluid and woken at night to drink. Of late he has been increasingly lethargic and has lost his appetite. There is no other significant past medical history. His sister has spina bifida and is wheelchair bound.

On examination his weight and height were on the 0.4th centile and his Tanner staging was P_4G_4. He was pale with marked genu valgum. He was normotensive. He had a grade 1/6 ejection systolic murmur, heard maximally over the lower left sternal edge.

Serum sodium	142 mmol/l
Serum potassium	5.1 mmol/l
Serum calcium	2.42 mmol/l
Serum phosphate	3.0 mmol/l
Serum alkaline phosphatase	211 IU/l
Serum parathormone	1425 pg/ml (normal 12–81 pg/ml)

1. What is the cause of his genu valgum?
2. What is the most likely underlying diagnosis?
3. Give a further investigation to confirm the underlying diagnosis.

QUESTION 17.4

A 35-week infant boy is noted to be jaundiced at 12 hours of age. He was born by normal vaginal delivery, with membranes rupturing 14 hours previously. Antenatally there had been a threatened miscarriage at 12 weeks, otherwise his mother, a Thai woman, had been well.

Haemoglobin	13.4 g/dl
White cell count	$6.4 \times 10^9/l$
Platelets	$104 \times 10^9/l$
Serum bilirubin	146 μmol/l
Maternal blood group	O positive
Infant blood group	B positive
Direct Coombs test	positive

A double-volume exchange transfusion is performed at 18 hours of age. Following transfusion, his haemoglobin is 17.8 g/dl. Six days later, he is noted to be more jaundiced. He is on total parenteral nutrition (120 ml/kg) and nil orally, as he has not tolerated enteral feeds. He has been afebrile.

Haemoglobin	17.2 g/dl
White cell count	$12.2 \times 10^9/l$
Platelets	$234 \times 10^9/l$
Total bilirubin	323 μmol/l
Conjugated bilirubin	221 μmol/l
Serum aspartate transaminase	64 IU/l (normal 10–45 IU/l)
Serum gamma glutamyl transferase	2 IU/l (normal <200 IU/l)
Serum alkaline phosphatase	223 IU/l (normal 150–700 IU/l)
Serum albumin	37 g/l
TORCH screen	negative
Thyroid function tests	normal

Alpha-1-antitryspin phenotype	MM
Urinary reducing substances	negative

1. What is the diagnosis?
2. What investigations would you do?
3. What four management steps would you initiate?

QUESTION 17.5

A 21-month-old boy was referred to the clinic because of delayed speech development. He had been born at term following a normal pregnancy. Delivery had been by Caesarean section because of a non-reassuring fetal heart rate pattern but he was breathing spontaneously by 4 minutes after a brief period of mask ventilation. The parents had taken him to the health visitor because he was still not saying anything comprehensible, in contrast to his older sister who was speaking in sentences at this stage. They thought he understood most simple things that were said to him and he would, for instance, go and pick up a ball if asked to. He had smiled at 5 weeks, rolled over at 4 months and was sitting unsupported by 10 months. He did not crawl (neither had his father) but was walking round the furniture at a year of age and walking unaided by 15 months. He was said to be a little clumsy. He had passed his health visitor hearing screen at 9 months. There had been no developmental stasis or regression. The parents were unrelated and had one healthy older girl. A maternal uncle had been told he had a rare blood disorder, otherwise there was no significant family history.

On examination he was well, alert and interested in his surroundings. He scored appropriately for his age on Griffiths developmental assessment scales for personal/social, eye/hand coordination and performance but was 6 months behind on the hearing/speech scale and 3 months behind on the locomotor scale. Neurological examination revealed a rather broad-based gait and a pronounced lordosis. General clinical examination revealed no abnormalities.

1. What diagnosis do you most wish to exclude?
2. Give one simple test that would allow you to do this.

Paper 17 *Answers*

17

ANSWER 17.1

1. Small heart
   Diffuse peribronchial infiltrates/thickening
   Right pleural effusion
   Hyperinflated lungs (flat diaphragm)
2. Obstructed infradiaphragmatic anomalous venous connection

The time course of this patient's illness suggests a congenital cardiac lesion. The principal radiological features of a small heart with pulmonary (interstitial) oedema support the diagnosis of obstructed anomalous venous connection.

ANSWER 17.2

1. Pulmonary haemosiderosis
2. Examination of sputum for haemosiderin-laden macrophages
3. Oxygen for hypoxaemia
   Bronchodilators may provide symptomatic relief
   Steroids and azathioprine have been employed but with uncertain effect

Pulmonary haemosiderosis is an uncommon disorder characterised by recurrent alveolar haemorrhage. In children pulmonary haemosiderosis occurs largely as a primary phenomenon, whereas in adults it tends to complicate another underlying illness such as cardiac disease or collagen vascular disease. Patients with primary pulmonary haemosiderosis may be further classified into four groups: those with accompanying glomerulonephritis (Goodpasture's syndrome – extremely rare in childhood); those with cows' milk protein sensitivity; those with associated cardiac or pancreatic disease (myocarditis, pancreatic insufficiency); and those with idiopathic disease.

Most primary pulmonary haemosiderosis is idiopathic. This disorder occurs most frequently in the first decade of life. Cases are distributed equally among males and females. Clinically, the process is characterised by the acute or insidious onset of pulmonary symptoms including cough, haemoptysis, wheezing, cyanosis and dyspnoea. Haematemesis may occur as a

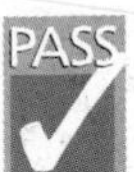

result of swallowed pulmonary blood. Other common findings include pallor from anaemia, poor weight gain and fatigue.

The aetiology is unknown. It is accompanied by iron-deficiency anaemia and haemosiderin deposition in the lung tissues. It presents with respiratory features of haemoptysis, tachypnoea and wheeze. There may be in addition failure to thrive and iron-deficiency anaemia. The chest radiograph varies according to the state of disease at the time. The radiological signs may precede the clinical symptoms. There is a generalised interstitial shadowing, which may be interspersed with areas of collapse and atelectasis. These areas are seen following haemorrhage and may extend rapidly after a haemorrhage.

Diagnosis rests on finding haemosiderin-laden macrophages in sputum. Treatment of pulmonary haemosiderosis is largely supportive. Patients with acute pulmonary haemorrhage may require oxygen or mechanical ventilation and blood transfusion. Steroids, with or without other immunosuppressants, may be used in treatment but desferrioxamine has been used with variable results. A milk-free diet may be beneficial in infants with cows' milk sensitivity. The outcome is variable but usually one of disease progression. Death may occur early following a massive pulmonary haemorrhage or the patient may survive into adulthood and develop fibrosing alveolitis.

ANSWER 17.3

1. Renal osteodystrophy
2. Bilateral renal dysplasia
3. Ultrasound scan of the renal tract

Renal dysplasia is defined as the abnormal qualitative development of the renal parenchyma. It is not a single entity but a spectrum of malformations. This boy has diffuse bilateral dysplasia, which is usually inherited in a sporadic fashion. It can be also associated with congenital urinary obstruction. It causes a gradual reduction in renal function during life and often there is a urinary concentrating defect because the collecting ducts are affected. There is a wide spectrum of clinical severity in such cases. The diagnosis can be confirmed histologically but is usually suggested by the ultrasound appearances of the parenchyma.

This boy had end-stage renal failure secondary to renal dysplasia. He had short stature also as a consequence of this condition. His polydipsia is because of his poor urinary concentrating ability and his recent deterioration relates to his worsening renal function. He had a marked anaemia of chronic disease that caused his flow murmur.

ANSWER 17.4

1. Inspissated bile syndrome
2. Assess stool for pigment
   Abdominal ultrasound
   Urine microscopy

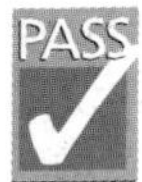

3. Increase fluid volume
   Persist in trying to establish enteral feeds
   Start a choleretic – ursodeoxycholic acid
   Consideration of an early surgical opinion

This infant has inspissated bile syndrome secondary to haemolytic disease and a degree of dehydration. Other causes of conjugated hyperbilirubinaemia need to be considered, particularly obstructive causes. It is also important to screen for an occult urinary tract infection. The initial management should include liberalisation of fluids, and encouragement of bile flow with enteral feeds and the use of ursodeoxycholic acid. A surgical opinion should be considered if there is no clinical improvement.

ANSWER 17.5

1. Duchenne muscular dystrophy
2. Serum creatine phosphokinase

Duchenne dystrophy is an X-linked recessive condition arising from an abnormality of the dystrophin gene (usually deletion) at the Xp21.2 locus. Affected boys (the condition has also been reported in association with Turner's syndrome) develop progressive muscular weakness and die from respiratory failure in the second to third decade. Early motor development is usually normal although hypotonia and mildly delayed motor development may occur. The typical pseudohypertrophy of the calves is not usually apparent until after the second year and Gower's sign may not be present until after 3 years of age. Boys with Duchenne dystrophy are significantly more likely to have speech delay than the general population and this may be a presenting feature that distracts attention from the true underlying diagnosis. Other features are cardiomyopathy and some degree of intellectual impairment. Definitive diagnosis is by muscle histochemistry. There is no specific treatment.

Paper 18 *Questions*

18

QUESTION 18.1

A male infant is born at 30 weeks' gestation, birthweight 1340 g, following a placental abruption. He is intubated at birth and develops a right-sided pneumothorax, which is successfully drained. He requires ventilation for a further 4 days, is extubated onto nasal CPAP for a further 48 hours and is out of oxygen by 7 days of age. He remains well for the following 2 weeks before developing tachypnoea, recession and an oxygen requirement (35%) in association with a period of temperature instability. His parents both have upper respiratory tract infections.

Haemoglobin	9.7 g/dl
White blood count	$6.1 \times 10^9/l$
Platelets	$225 \times 10^9/l$

He is transfused, blood cultures are taken and he is commenced on antibiotics. A chest radiograph is performed (Fig. 18.1).

1. What does the chest radiograph show?
2. How would you confirm the diagnosis?
3. What are the therapeutic options? List two.

QUESTION 18.2

A previously healthy 9-year-old boy is referred to outpatients by his GP. On three occasions his parents have been woken by noises emanating from his bedroom. On two occasions things had stopped when they reached his bedroom but on the last occasion he was seen to have repetitive twitching of the right side of his face. At 15 months he had one febrile convulsion but has no other medical history of note. His father recalls being teased about 'mild epilepsy' when he started secondary school. On examination the boy is well; height and weight are on the 50th centile for his age. His head circumference is 0.5 cm above the 90th centile. He is normotensive and cardiorespiratory examination is normal. There are no neurocutaneous stigmata and neurological examination is entirely normal.

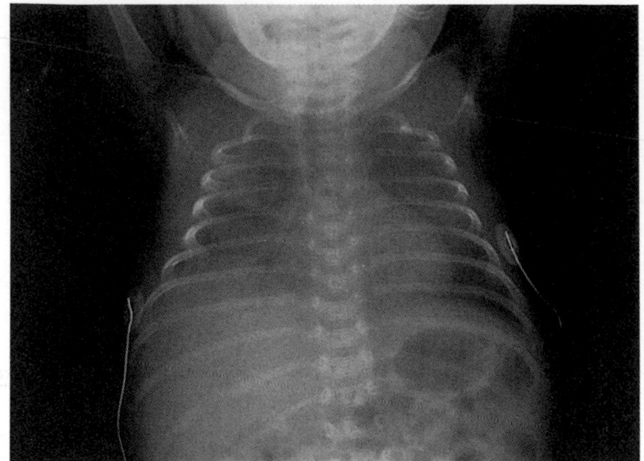

Fig. 18.1

1. What is the likely diagnosis?
2. What investigation would you perform?
3. What is the prognosis?
4. Would you begin any treatment? If so what would you start?

QUESTION 18.3

A 3-year-old girl presented with her first generalised seizure. She had previously been well but had severe behavioural problems. Her grandmother cared for her during the day and commented that her granddaughter always needed to have something in her mouth, such as a pacifier or a bottle. Very recently attempts were made to wean her off the pacifier. She suffered a head injury in her father's care 2 weeks previously but reportedly did not lose consciousness. The child was on no medication. There was no significant family history other than her father's alcoholism.

On examination she was postictal, having been treated with rectal diazepam, which had terminated the fit. She had not received intravenous fluids. There were no focal neurological signs and her reflexes were globally reduced with equivocal plantar responses. She had slightly full peripheral pulses. Her blood pressure was 80/45 mmHg and her heart rate 70 beats per minute. Heart sounds were normal. Abdominal examination was unremarkable. No bruising was noted.

Serum sodium	121 mmol/l
Serum potassium	2.7 mmol/l
Serum urea	1.7 mmol/l
Serum creatinine	24 µmol/l
Blood glucose	3.8 mmol/l
Serum osmolality	253 mosmol/kg
Haemoglobin	8.9 g/dl
White blood count	$4.8 \times 10^9/l$
Platelets	$209 \times 10^9/l$
Haematocrit	25%

Urine sodium	5 mmol/l
Urine creatinine	800 μmol/l
Urine osmolality	<100 mosmol/kg
Urine dipstick and microscopy	normal
Urine toxicology screen	normal

Following urinary catheterisation she passed 30 ml/kg/hour of urine.

1. Suggest the cause of this girl's electrolyte abnormalities.
2. What is the immediate management?

QUESTION 18.4

A 14-year-old girl presents with a 3-week history of malaise, anorexia and progressive jaundice. She has been vomiting persistently for 24 hours before admission. She is in foster care and presently is under the care of the child psychiatry department because of behavioural problems. She is not on any current medication. Her mother is a registered drug addict. On examination, she is drowsy and has slurred speech. She has bilateral palmar erythema and icteric sclerae. Multiple spider naevi are noted on her anterior chest wall. On palpation of her abdomen, she has firm hepatomegaly and splenomegaly, 2 cm and 4 cm below their respective costal margins.

Haemoglobin	$11.0 \times 10^9/l$
White cell count	$5.4 \times 10^9/l$
Platelets	$20 \times 10^9/l$
Blood glucose	1.2 mmol/l
Serum protein	77 g/l
Serum albumin	29 g/l
Serum bilirubin	113 μmol/l
Alanine transaminase	4001 IU/l
Prothrombin time	21 s (control 10–12 s) (not significantly correctable with vitamin K and fresh frozen plasma)
Activated partial thromboplastin time	53 s (control 24–36 s)
IgG	19.2 g/l (normal 5–16 g/l)
IgM	1.3 g/l (normal 0.5–2.2 g/l)
IgA	2.1 g/l (normal 0.7–4.0 g/l)
Coombs test	negative
Hepatitis serology	negative
Urinary copper (post penicillamine)	slightly elevated

1. What is the diagnosis?
2. What is the most likely cause?
3. What is the management?

QUESTION 18.5

A 2-year-old West Indian boy was admitted to hospital with a 2-day history of a limp associated with a painful, swollen left ankle and fever. He had been born in the UK. Both parents were hospital workers. On examination he was moderately unwell with a temperature of 38.9°C. The left ankle was red, hot, swollen and tender, particularly over the lateral malleolus and lower fibula. A radiograph was reported as showing some soft-tissue swelling but no bony abnormality. The ankle was explored and at operation some necrotic bone was removed. Purulent-looking material failed to grow anything on culture and blood cultures were negative. He was treated with flucloxacillin for 3 weeks.

Over the next 2 months he continued to have pain in the left ankle and to run an intermittent fever, in spite of a series of antibiotic regimens. At the end of this time he was admitted to a different hospital with a 5-day history of becoming lethargic and progressively less well. On examination he was pyrexial and wasted. The left leg was encased in plaster of Paris; radiography showed partial destruction of the metaphysis and epiphysis of the fibula with periosteal reaction and new bone formation.

CSF microscopy	137 white cells/mm^3 (99% mononuclear) no organisms seen on Gram stain
CSF protein	3 g/l
CSF glucose	<1 mmol/l
Blood glucose	6.4 mmol/l
Tuberculin skin test	no induration or redness

1. What is the most likely diagnosis?
2. What other clinical signs would you look for?
3. List two investigations you would perform.

Paper 18 *Answers*

18

ANSWER 18.1

1. Raised right hemi-diaphragm – probable eventration
2. Ultrasound to look at diaphragmatic movement
3. No treatment if no respiratory problems
   Plication if required

Eventration of the diaphragm is relatively rare. The muscle is permanently elevated but retains its continuity and attachments to the costal margin. It may be caused by a phrenic nerve injury or a congenital muscular deficiency of the diaphragm. Clinical manifestations are diverse, varying from mild gastrointestinal symptoms and tachypnoea to severe respiratory distress requiring ventilation. Ultrasound may be used to ascertain whether diaphragmatic movement is limited but appropriate. Plication of the affected hemi-diaphragm will reduce symptoms and is thought to improve the potential for lung growth. Its role in asymptomatic patients is controversial.

ANSWER 18.2

1. Benign Rolandic epilepsy
2. An electroencephalogram (EEG), which should show centrotemporal spikes (Rolandic area)
3. Good – spontaneous remission usually occurs before 15–16 years of age
4. Treatment is tailored to the needs of the individual and his family. The overall benign nature of the seizures and eventual good outcome allow for possible expectant management without anticonvulsants in most cases. Recurrent seizures, and sometimes parental pressure, may necessitate treatment in which case carbamazepine is the first line choice

Benign Rolandic epilepsy (benign partial epilepsy with centrotemporal spikes) is an epileptic syndrome characterised by simple partial seizures with motor and somatosensory symptoms confined to the face and extremities. It is defined by the International Classification of Epilepsy as an idiopathic localisation-related epileptic syndrome, no underlying cause, localised origin of seizure, usually idiopathic with no underlying structural lesions.

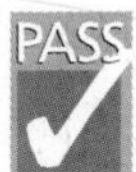

It most commonly presents at night in a 9–10-year-old boy who suddenly wakes up 2–3 hours after falling asleep. The seizure lasts 1–3 minutes and is characterised by guttural sounds, unilateral twitching of facial muscles and unintelligible speech. Seizures are largely simple partial seizures (80%) with focal motor or, less commonly, somatosensory phenomena. But some children may have generalised tonic–clonic seizures. The EEG is usually characteristic although the diagnosis can usually be made from the history. Neuroimaging is unnecessary. Spontaneous resolution occurs in over 75% by 15–16 years of age.

ANSWER 18.3

1. Excess water intake (water intoxication)
2. Severe fluid restriction

This young girl has acute water intoxication, a rare cause of hyponatraemia in childhood. As her pacifier was withdrawn she was given many more bottles of tap water, which she drank voraciously day and night. Water intoxication is usually seen in adolescents with emotional or psychiatric problems. She had mild clinical signs of volume overload, a low plasma and urine osmolality (with all electrolyte levels reduced), a reduced haematocrit and voided very large quantities of urine. Her fractional excretion of sodium (FENa) was 0.1% and a FENa of <1% suggests that her kidneys are compensating for the hyponatraemia and are avidly retaining sodium. The intake or administration of large quantities of hypotonic liquid is the only explanation for these findings. Fluid restriction, in order to increase the plasma sodium gradually, is standard first-line treatment. Intravenous 0.9% saline is used only if further hyponatraemic seizures occur.

She does not have the syndrome of inappropriate antidiuretic hormone secretion (SIADH). This case shares a number of features with SIADH such as hyponatraemia and a low plasma osmolality; however, in SIADH there is usually an inappropriately elevated urine osmolality, a reduced urine output and a urine sodium concentration in excess of 20 mmol/l (as renal sodium handling is normal in SIADH and is governed by the sodium intake).

ANSWER 18.4

1. Acute liver failure on the background of chronic liver disease
2. Autoimmune hepatitis
3. Treatment with steroids

This child presents in acute liver failure and the initial management is directed at this with multi-organ support and early anticipation of any hepatic or neurological deterioration. This includes fluid restriction, maintenance of normoglycaemia, broad-spectrum antibiotic and antifungal coverage and coagulation support. An acetylcysteine infusion at maintenance dose should also be started. This girl is showing the stigmata of chronic liver disease. Her hypergammaglobulinaemia and negative Coombs test make autoimmune hepatitis more likely than Wilson's disease. Positive autoantibody screening (antineutrophil, smooth muscle and liver–kidney–microsomal antibodies) will help support the diagnosis. As liver biopsy is contraindicated (due to the coagulopathy), management with steroids must be started immediately. A confirmatory biopsy can be done at a later date.

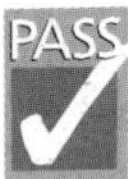

ANSWER 18.5

1. Miliary tuberculosis with tuberculous osteomyelitis and probable meningitis
2. Choroidal tubercles
3. Chest radiograph
   Exploration and culture of osteomyelitic lesion

Generalised cachexia associated with chronic fever and cough unresponsive to conventional antibiotic therapy is highly suspicious of a low-grade infective process such as tuberculosis. Alternative diagnoses include autoimmune diseases and malignancy or tropical diseases such as filariasis. The fact that both parents work in hospital makes exposure to tuberculosis a possibility even if there is no history. The negative skin test is classical of miliary disease. This boy had choroidal tubercles on fundoscopy and miliary shadowing on the chest radiograph. Acid–alcohol-fast bacilli were seen on fluorescent microscopy. He was treated with rifampicin, isoniazid, pyrazinamide and ethambutol until sensitivities were known. Treatment with the first three were continued for a year as osteomyelitis is often more refractory to treatment.

Paper 19 *Questions*

19

QUESTION 19.1

An 8-year-old boy is referred with a history of faecal soiling. He was born at term after an uneventful pregnancy and delivery. He passed meconium within 24 hours of birth. No problems were noticed by his parents until attempts at potty training failed and he subsequently failed to achieve faecal continence. There were no associated urinary problems. He had also had a long-term history of otitis media, chronically perforated tympanic membranes and poor language development. He was generally felt to be progressing poorly at school and disliked physical activities. There had also been periodic concerns raised by Social Services with regard to the family dynamics since his mother had remarried. His maternal uncle, who had a long-standing history of depression and alcohol abuse, had recently moved into the family home.

He was very reluctant to be examined. He appeared to have a flat affect and seemed to be breathing through his mouth. He was appropriately grown. Rectal examination revealed a wide, gaping anus with fissuring and a flattened posterior anal margin and soft stool in the rectum. In view of the findings the family were again assessed by Social Services who concluded that there was no evidence of sexual abuse. Attempts to alleviate the problem with aggressive laxative therapy failed and a referral was made to the Child Psychiatry service.

1. Suggest two causes for the patient's soiling.
2. What investigations would you perform? List two.

QUESTION 19.2

A 9-year-old girl with hereditary spherocytosis is referred by her GP. Typically she has a haemoglobin of 10–11 g/dl, and a reticulocyte count of 10%. Over the last 3 days she has become very tired and irritable. On examination she is noted to be pale. She has a tachycardia and systolic murmur. There is no hepatomegaly but splenomegaly is evident. On further enquiries her mother says the girl has had a viral-like illness with fever, malaise, URTI symptoms and conjunctivitis. Her younger sister had a similar illness 2 weeks previously and still has a diffuse macular red rash on the trunk and proximal extremities (both arms and legs). The rash is more prominent on the extensor surfaces; the soles and palms are spared but the rash is said be itchy. A similar rash had appeared on her face but had disappeared.

Haemoglobin	3.7 g/dl
White cell count	$8.4 \times 10^9/l$
Neutrophils	$0.4 \times 10^9/l$
Lymphocytes	$7.9 \times 10^9/l$
Platelets	$104 \times 10^9/l$
Reticulocytes	0.4%

1. What is the emergency here?
2. What is its aetiology?
3. How can you confirm this?
4. How would you manage this girl?
5. What is the prognosis?

QUESTION 19.3

Following a pregnancy complicated by gestational diabetes, a female infant was delivered at 34 weeks' gestation by emergency Caesarean section because of fetal distress in labour. She weighed 2150 g. Her initial condition was poor and she required ventilatory support for respiratory distress syndrome. On day 2 macroscopic haematuria was noted. On examination a palpable right-sided abdominal mass was discovered.

Serum sodium	128 mmol/l
Serum potassium	7.5 mmol/l
Serum urea	18.0 mmol/l
Serum creatinine	212 µmol/l
Serum bicarbonate	17 mmol/l
Blood glucose	2.8 mmol/l
Serum aspartate transaminase	12 IU/l (normal 10–45 IU/l)
Serum alanine transaminase	6 IU/l (normal 0–25 IU/l)
Serum gamma glutamyl transferase	23 IU/l (normal <200 IU/l)
Haemoglobin	12.1 g/dl
White blood count	$8.8 \times 10^9/l$
Platelets	$47 \times 10^9/l$
Urine dipstick	+++ blood, ++ protein

Ultrasound scanning of the renal tract revealed a large right kidney and normal-appearing left kidney. Doppler studies demonstrated poor blood flow within the right kidney and normal flow within the left. There was no evidence of thrombosis in the renal veins or inferior vena cava.

1. What is the diagnosis?
2. How would you treat this condition?
3. What six further investigations would further define the underlying aetiology?

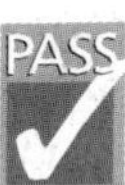

QUESTION 19.4

A 6-year-old boy is admitted with a 3-week history of progressive non-bilious projectile vomiting. His mother states that he has also had diarrhoea associated with some specks of fresh blood over the last 2 months. She feels her son has lost a significant amount of weight. In the past he was admitted at 4 years of age with staphylococcal pneumonia and has also required incision and drainage of two cervical lymph node abscesses. He has a sister who is well. On examination he is pale, not clubbed. His weight is below the 2nd centile and his height is on the 9th centile. He is 7.5% dehydrated. His chest is clinically clear. He has normal heart sounds. His BP is 90/68 mmHg. His upper abdomen is distended with visible peristalsis and a succussion splash. There is no tenderness on palpation, or hepatomegaly. Gentle perianal examination shows a deep anal fissure.

Haemoglobin	9.2 g/dl
White cell count	12.4×10^9/l
Platelets	556×10^9/l
MCV	69.3 fl
ESR	45 mm/h
Serum sodium	136 mmol/l
Serum potassium	2.7 mmol/l
Serum chloride	87 mmol/l
Serum bicarbonate	27 mmol/l
Serum urea	13.2 mmol/l
Serum creatinine	66 μmol/l
Serum albumin	34 g/l
Alanine transaminase	24 IU/l (normal 2–53 IU/l)
Serum bilirubin	7 μmol/l
Alkaline phosphatase	213 IU/l
C-reactive protein	102 mg/l
Serum immunoglobulins	normal
Ig G subclasses	normal
Lymphocyte subsets	normal
Sweat chloride	33 mmol/120 g
Chest radiograph	normal

1. What further investigations would you perform? List eight.
2. What is the diagnosis?
3. What is the treatment for the immediate problem?
4. What is the long-term management?

QUESTION 19.5

A 14-year-old girl was seen in clinic with a history of amenorrhoea and headache. Menarche occurred normally at 12 years and she had developed a normal menstrual cycle. Nine months before her clinic visit she had had a flu-like illness. Following this her periods became more scanty and her last period had occurred 4 months previously. During this time she had had

frontal headaches and became increasingly tired. The headache and tiredness were most marked in the afternoon but were present throughout the day. She had become constipated and was increasingly disinterested in going to school. This last problem was partly a result of waking during the night and feeling tired the following morning. Her appetite had decreased but she did not think she had lost weight. She was an only child. Her father had recently left home and she lived with her mother. There were no illnesses in the family apart from a first cousin with type 1 diabetes.

On examination she had a somewhat flat affect, appeared lethargic and was slow to answer questions. Her height was on the 10th centile and weight on the 50th. Pulse rate was 64/min, blood pressure 110/60 and temperature normal. Full clinical examination revealed no other obvious abnormalities.

1. Give two possible diagnoses which might explain the girl's symptoms.
2. List three investigations you would perform.

Paper 19 *Answers*

19

ANSWER 19.1

1. Myotonic dystrophy
   Hirschsprung's disease
2. Rectal biopsy
   PCR, looking for trinucleotide repeat expansion at the myotonic dystrophy locus

It is clearly essential to exclude a diagnosis of Hirschsprung's disease by rectal biopsy, although the history here is not typical. In retrospect this boy's poor school performance and dislike of physical activities were directly related to his myotonic dystrophy and his apparent mouth-breathing was a result of myopathic facies. Myopathic involvement of smooth as well as striated muscle is well recognised in patients with myotonic dystrophy. Abnormalities of smooth muscle lead to disordered gastrointestinal motility with megaoesophagus (resulting in dysphagia and dyspepsia) and megacolon. Incontinence is rare, but if it occurs in children the features may mimic those of sexual abuse. It is thought that there are atrophic and neural as well as myopathic factors involved in the pathological process. These abnormalities produce a decrease in resting pressure in the anal canal and a reflex myotonic contraction subsequent to rectal distension.

ANSWER 19.2

1. Acute aplastic anaemia
2. Parvovirus B19 infection in a patient affected by chronic haemolytic anaemia
3. Parvovirus B19 IgM or viral DNA detection using PCR technique
4. Supportive measures to reduce cardiorespiratory compromise
   Intravenous immunoglobulin
5. Good – spontaneous recovery occurs

Parvovirus B19 was not associated with a disease until 1981, when it was found to be associated with an aplastic crisis in a patient with sickle-cell anaemia. It was then discovered to cause other illnesses – fifth disease

(erythema infectiosum or slapped cheek disease), intrauterine infection leading to severe anaemia and hydrops fetalis and some forms of acute arthritis.

Parvovirus B19 replicates in erythroid progenitor cells. This inhibits erythropoiesis, leading to a transient anaemia in healthy individuals, but may cause chronic anaemia (in immunodeficient patients) and an aplastic crisis (in patients with chronic haemolytic anaemias). Treatment of the aplastic crisis is largely supportive, with transfusions and general cardiorespiratory support. Intravenous immunoglobulin has been shown in some cases to reduce the duration of the course and may be of value, particularly in immunocompromised patients. If the infection is acquired by a seronegative woman, there is a 9–10% risk of fetal hydrops or death in the first 20 weeks of pregnancy. This is less if infection is acquired in the second half of pregnancy.

ANSWER 19.3

1. Bilateral renal venous thrombosis
2. Intravenous heparin infusion
   Correction of hyperkalaemia (salbutamol, bicarbonate, glucose and insulin infusions)
   Acute peritoneal dialysis
3. Blood culture
   Haematocrit
   Protein C assay
   Protein S assay
   Factor V Leiden assay
   Assessment for prothrombin 20210GA and/or methylenetetrahydrofolate reductase mutations

This baby has acute renal failure and therefore must have bilateral renal involvement. Unilateral renal venous thrombosis (RVT) does not reduce overall renal function. Normal blood flow in the renal vein does not exclude RVT as the thrombus initially develops in the intrarenal venous radicals and may not extend to impede renal vein flow. Similarly, despite intrarenal thrombus formation, the ultrasound appearances of the renal parenchyma and the Doppler blood flow within the kidney may be normal. Regarding treatment, there is debate as to the efficacy of anticoagulants in these circumstances and some authorities advocate a conservative, supportive approach.

ANSWER 19.4

1. Nitrotetrazolium blue test
   Neutrophil oxidative burst testing
   Flow cytometric assay of white blood cells
   Flow cytometric assay of mother's white blood cells
   Abdominal ultrasound
   Barium meal and follow-through
   White cell scan
   Endoscopy/colonoscopy with serial biopsies

2. Chronic granulomatous disease with functional pyloric stenosis and colitis
3. Intravenous rehydration
   Nasogastric tube and free drainage
   Oral or intravenous steroids for the granulomatous pyloric obstruction
4. Prophylactic trimethoprim and itraconazole
   Nutritional support
   5-aminosalcyclic acid
   Multi-specialist support

Chronic granulomatous disease is due to a defect in the respiratory burst in white cells. Patients will present with either recurrent infections, particularly with catalase producing bacteria, or chronic inflammation. The gut is commonly involved and the patient may have obstructive granulomatous lesions such as pyloric stenosis or oesphageal stricture or a colitis that mimics Crohn's disease. These lesions respond to steroid treatment though they can re-occur. Siblings can be screened in the neonatal period.

ANSWER 19.5

1. Hypothyroidism
   Depression
2. Thyroid function tests
   Bone age
   CT head scan

This girl's investigations showed a serum free T_4 of 5 pmol/l, a TSH of 150 IU/l, a bone age of 12 years and a CT brain scan was normal. These findings are diagnostic of acquired hypothyroidism. After treatment with thyroxine her periods returned, her growth accelerated and her mood and affect returned to normal. The most likely aetiology of the hypothyroidism is lymphocytic (Hashimoto's) thyroiditis, which typically occurs in teenage girls and may become symptomatic following a viral illness. This supposition is strengthened by the occurrence of another autoimmune disease in the family and confirmed by the presence of antiperoxidase antibodies in the patient's serum. There is often a latent phase during which lymphocytic infiltration causes a goitre but no clinical symptoms. It is important to exclude an intracranial space-occupying lesion as a cause for her headaches and mood change.

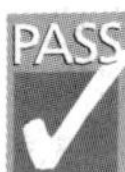

Paper 20 *Questions*

20

QUESTION 20.1

A 9-month-old Bangladeshi boy presents with a 1-day history of fever, poor feeding and irritability. His parents have noticed that he is prone to be 'chesty' and wheezes intermittently in association with upper respiratory tract infections. He was born at term, birthweight 3600 g, being the second child of healthy parents who are distant cousins. He was admitted to the neonatal unit on the first day of life with a hoarse cry, hypoglycaemia and hypotonia. He was found to have a laryngeal web. His hypoglycaemia resolved but he continued to feed poorly for some time. He had a previous admission at the age of 2 months with several brief focal seizures with associated EEG changes but a normal CT head scan. He was commenced on anticonvulsants at that time. A heart murmur was also noted during that admission and an atrial septal defect identified on echocardiogram. Developmentally he smiled at 8 weeks of age. He is not yet sitting unsupported. On examination he is febrile (39°C). Both eardrums are pink and his throat is injected. He dislikes being handled and an infection screen is performed.

Haemoglobin	9.4 g/dl
White cell count	$5.7 \times 10^9/l$
Neutrophils	$4.6 \times 10^9/l$
Lymphocytes	$0.3 \times 10^9/l$
Monocytes	$0.7 \times 10^9/l$
Eosinophils	$0.1 \times 10^9/l$
Platelets	$342 \times 10^9/l$
Blood film	microcytic, hypochromic
Serum sodium	135 mmol/l
Serum potassium	4.2 mmol/l
Serum urea	3.1 mmol/l
Serum creatinine	65 μmol/l
Serum calcium	2.05 mmol/l
CSF microscopy	no cells, no organisms seen on Gram stain
CSF glucose	normal
CSF protein	normal
Blood cultures	sterile
Chest radiograph	normal

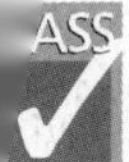

He makes an uneventful recovery; no cause for his acute illness is identified.

1. How would you investigate this child's problems further? (List five.)
2. Suggest a diagnosis.

QUESTION 20.2

A 6-year-old girl has been under follow-up for seizures for the previous 8 months. She had presented at that time with a generalised tonic clonic seizure and was started on sodium valproate. This failed to control the seizures and after 2 months carbamazepine was started. Since then the seizures have become mixed in pattern, with tonic–clonic episodes, absences, myoclonic jerks and partial motor seizures. She is the second child of healthy unrelated parents and her development to date had been normal. She has been otherwise well, although her parents feel she has become unsteady, leading to several falls. On examination she is tremulous and ataxic. Deep tendon reflexes are brisk with evidence of ankle clonus. Her EEG on admission shows a disorganised background and bursts of spikes and slow waves. Large amplitude waves are produced in the occipital region on phototic stimulation.

Electro-retinogram	isoelectric
Visual evoked responses	distorted, high-amplitude response

1. What is the likely diagnosis?
2. How would you establish the diagnosis?
3. What is the prognosis?

QUESTION 20.3

A 5-year-old boy was admitted to the orthopaedic ward with a limp and a painful right hip. On examination there was limitation of internal rotation of the right hip. A hip radiograph showed only soft tissue swelling around the affected joint. He was afebrile. A diagnosis of transient synovitis of the hip was made. He was treated with bed rest, ibuprofen and traction.

Haemoglobin	12.7 g/dl
White cell count	4.3×10^9/l
Platelets	307×10^9/l
ESR	6 mm/h
Serum sodium	141 mmol/l
Serum potassium	4.3 mmol/l
Serum urea	3.6 mmol/l
Serum creatinine	42 μmol/l

His symptoms settled completely. Just before discharge a week later he developed of a pruritic rash and complained of feeling hot. On examination he had a fleeting urticarial rash and a temperature of 38.0°C. No other abnormalities were noted. The following day he was tired and lethargic and had little interest in food. He remained febrile but his rash had settled. His blood pressure was normal. His blood tests were repeated:

Haemoglobin	11.9 g/dl
White cell count	5.6×10^9/l
Platelets	289×10^9/l
ESR	8 mm/h
Serum sodium	141 mmol/l
Serum potassium	5.8 mmol/l
Serum urea	27.1 mmol/l
Serum creatinine	199 μmol/l
Urine dipstick	++ blood, + protein
Urine microscopy	many red blood cells and eosinophils, no casts, no other elements

1. What is the cause of this boy's renal impairment?
2. What has precipitated the problem?
3. Give three other causes.

QUESTION 20.4

A 2-year-old-year girl is rushed into the Accident and Emergency department with respiratory difficulties. She is drowsy, cyanosed and has a respiratory rate of 12/min. There is marked sternal and subcostal recession, and a harsh stridor is audible. Her father explains that she has been unwell for 48 hours, with vomiting and watery diarrhoea. She has had sticky eyes today. She is normally fit and well but has not been immunised. On examination, her oxygen saturation in air is 84% and her temperature is 39.1°C. She is cool peripherally with a capillary refill time of 6 seconds, and a pulse rate of 140/min. She has a macular erythematous rash over her abdomen, a paronychia on her left thumb and old discoloured bruising over her shins. Palpation of her abdomen reveals generalised tenderness.

Haemoglobin	11.4 g/dl
White cell count	1.0×10^9/l
Neutrophils	0.4×10^9/l
Lymphocytes	0.3×10^9/l
Platelets	14×10^9/l
Prothrombin time	19 s (control 11–15 s)
Activated partial thromboplastin time	67 s (control 24–35 s)
Serum sodium	133 mmol/l
Serum potassium	2.5 mmol/l
Serum chloride	93 mmol/l
Serum urea	7.8 mmol/l
Serum creatinine	62 μmol/l

1. What is the diagnosis?
2. List four other investigations.
3. What is the management of this child?

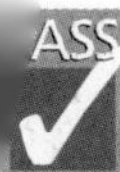

QUESTION 20.5

A 14-year-old boy was admitted to another hospital with a 3-month history of headache. For the 10 days prior to admission the headaches had become more severe and were associated with vomiting. During this time he had had a sore throat and earache. He had been treated with amoxicillin without effect and then co-trimoxazole, pizotifen and co-codamol. He had a past history of asthma for which he took inhaled steroids and a bronchodilator. In recent months his teachers had been concerned that he had been involved with a group of children who were known to inhale solvents and he had missed lessons on a couple of occasions without any explanation. Immediately before transfer from the referring hospital he had a generalised convulsion, terminated with intravenous diazepam.

On examination he was conscious but ill and drowsy with a temperature of 38.4°C. The right tympanic membrane was dull and grey; the left was dull and red and appeared painful. There was an upper motor neurone left facial weakness and there was bilateral papilloedema. Examination was otherwise unremarkable.

1. What are the two most likely diagnoses?
2. List three investigations you would carry out to define the problem and establish its aetiology.

Paper 20
Answers

20

ANSWER 20.1

1. Lymphocyte subsets
   Extended proliferation studies
   Immunoglobulins and subsets
   Antibody responses to diphtheria, tetanus, and Hib
   Isohaemagglutinins
2. Di George syndrome (22q11 deletion)

This boy appears to have a problem with recurrent infections and needs further investigation to delineate the problem. The combination of a possible immune problem with developmental delay, hypocalcaemia and a cardiac lesion suggests the diagnosis of Di George syndrome. Atrial septal defects are reported although they are atypical; laryngeal web occurs in approximately 1% of children with the 22q11 deletion. Hypocalcaemia tends to resolve and only about 30% of patients continue to need calcium supplements.

ANSWER 20.2

1. Juvenile neuronal ceroid-lipofuscinosis (Batten disease)
2. White cell enzyme studies
3. Poor – progressive. Increasing mental impairment, seizure activity, dementia and death

Neuronal ceroid lipofuscinoses (NCL) are progressive encephalopathies. They affect approximately 1 in 12 500 people worldwide. NCL are divided into three autosomal recessive subtypes, all assigned to different chromosomal loci. Infantile NCL (Santavuori–Haltia disease) begins between about 6 and 24 months of age and progresses rapidly. Affected children fail to thrive and have abnormally small heads (microcephaly). Also typical are myoclonic jerks. Patients usually die before age 5.

Late infantile NCL (Jansky–Bielschowsky disease) begins between 2 and 4 years. The typical early signs are loss of muscle coordination (ataxia) and seizures that do not respond to drugs. This form progresses rapidly and ends in death between ages 8 and 12.

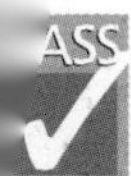

Juvenile NCL (Batten disease) usually appears between the ages of 5 and 10 years, when a previously normal child has begun to develop vision problems or seizures. In some cases the early signs are subtle, taking the form of personality and behaviour changes, slow learning, clumsiness or stumbling. The disease is progressive, with mental impairment, worsening seizures, and loss of sight and motor skills. Eventually, children with Batten disease become blind, bedridden and demented. Batten disease is often fatal by the late teens or twenties. There is no treatment for any of these conditions. Seizure control is attempted using anticonvulsant therapy but is difficult to achieve.

ANSWER 20.3

1. Acute tubulo-interstitial nephritis
2. Hypersensitivity reaction to ibuprofen
3. Other drugs (antibiotics, anti-inflammatory agents, anticonvulsants, diuretics)
   Infection (pyelonephritis)
   Immunological disorders (SLE, allograft rejection)

Acute tubulo-interstitial nephritis (TIN) is a relatively common cause of childhood acute renal impairment, with drug hypersensitivity the most frequently observed aetiology. Non-steroidal anti-inflammatory drugs are most often implicated. The onset of renal impairment, which may be mild or severe, is generally 1–8 weeks after exposure to the offending drug. The clinical picture is usually fever, rashes, fatigue and anorexia. Nephrotic syndrome is also occasionally seen. Microscopic haematuria, eosinophiluria and mild proteinuria are common. However, casts and macroscopic haematuria are seldom found. Frequently stopping the drug is all that is required to restore normal renal function.

ANSWER 20.4

1. Staphylococcal septicaemia and tracheitis leading to toxic shock syndrome
2. Blood culture
   Antistaphylolysin titres
   Swab from pus of paronychia
   Sputum or endotracheal secretions for Gram stain and culture after intubation
3. Primarily it is airway, breathing and circulation management, in that order. This child will need immediate intubation, preferably by a senior anaesthetist. Broad-spectrum antibiotics, including high-dose antistaphylococcal coverage. Complete drainage and irrigation of the infected site (paronychia in this case).

ANSWER 20.5

1. Cerebral abscess
   Cerebral tumour
2. Imaging of brain (CT or MR)
   Blood culture
   Exploration of mastoid

CT scan showed a typical rim-enhancing subdural empyema in the right frontal region with extension into the parietal region. The abscess was drained and the boy made an uneventful recovery. Exploration of the mastoid process revealed chronic mastoiditis. Extension of infection from the mastoid can occur either directly or as a result of a lateral sinus thrombophlebitis. It is a dangerous condition and carries a high subsequent morbidity. Treatment is with high-dose antibiotics and surgical drainage.

Index to questions